Leaping upon the Mountains

LEAPING
UPON
THE
MOUNTAINS

**Men Proclaiming Victory
over Sexual Child Abuse**

by Mike Lew

Foreword by Richard Hoffman

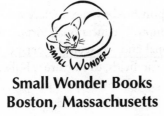

**Small Wonder Books
Boston, Massachusetts**

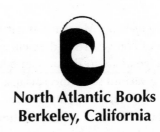

**North Atlantic Books
Berkeley, California**

Published by
Small Wonder Books
P.O. Box 1146
Jamaica Plain, MA 02130, U.S.A.
and
North Atlantic Books
P.O. Box 12327
Berkeley, CA 94712, U.S.A.

Book Design: Michael Woyton
Cover Design: Michael Mendelsohn at MM Design 2000, Inc.
Cover Art: © Photofusion by Paul Nagano
Author Photograph: © by Thom Harrigan

Printed in the United States of America.

Leaping upon the Mountains is partially sponsored by the Society for the Study of Native Arts and Sciences, a nonprofit educational corporation whose goals are to develop an educational and crosscultural perspective linking various scientific, social, and artistic fields; to nurture a holistic view of arts, sciences, humanities, and healing; and to publish and distribute literature on the relationship of mind, body, and nature.

CONTENTS

Acknowledgments   **ix**

Dedication   **xv**

Foreword by Richard Hoffman   **xix**

Introduction   **xxiii**

The Goal of *Leaping upon the Mountains*   **xxiv**

How I Went about It   **xxvii**

The Request for Resources   **xxxi**

The Responses   **xxxv**

Messages of Encouragement   **xxxix**

Unexpected Encouragement   **xliii**

A Reminder to the Reader   **xlvi**

Part One: Early Recovery   **1**

Books and Reading   **4**

Safe Environments   **9**

Professional Resources   **11**

Individual Counseling   **11**

Valuable Therapeutic Qualities   **14**

Group Therapy   **19**

A Person of Color:
Overcoming Barriers to Group Participation   **26**

Safe and Supportive Person(s)   **33**

Writing Activities   **42**

Other Creative Activities   **44**

Taking Difficult but Necessary Steps   **46**

Attention to Self   **49**

Attention to Others   **50**

Religion and Spirituality   50
Feelings   52
Intimate Relationships   53
Part Two: Mid–Recovery   55
Books and Reading   57
Safe Environments   61
Professional Resources   61
Safe and Supportive Person(s)   71
Writing Activities   76
Other Creative Activities   81
Taking Difficult but Necessary Steps   82
Attention to Self   84
Attention to Others   86
Religion and Spirituality   87
The Role of Feelings   88
Forgiveness, Risk, and Changes   89
Part Three: Late Recovery   91
Books and Reading   94
Safe Environments   95
Professional Resources   96
Safe and Supportive Persons   99
Writing Activities   105
Other Creative Activities   108
Taking Difficult but Necessary Steps   114
Confrontation   117
Limits and Boundaries   122
Attention to Self   125
Attention to Others   132
Religion and Spirituality   137
Interpersonal Exploration   140
Forgiveness   144
The Role of Feelings   144

Trust   **150**

Hope, Grace, and Moving On   **151**

**Part Four: Victorious Messages — Man to Man —
Argentina to Zimbabwe**   **155**

**Afterword — How Far We've Journeyed and
What Is Ahead**   **211**

Resources   **219**

Resource Bibliography   **219**

Other Resources   **227**

   World Wide Web Sites   **227**

   Organizations Listed Alphabetically by Countries **230**

About the Author   **267**

Acknowledgments

Many individuals contributed, directly and indirectly, to the creation of this book. Without their faith in the project and confidence in me — their steadfast support, encouragement, advice, concrete help, reality-testing, patience, good judgment and humor — *Leaping upon the Mountains* would never have been completed.

I thank my professional colleagues (many of whom have become valued friends) and my dear friends (many of whom have become unwitting colleagues). You all, in your individual ways, have been models of kindness, caring, loyalty, friendship, humanity, and love: Jim Acosta, Ayal Arnon, Janine Arseneau, Jon Arterton, Jeanne Axler, Euan Bear, Lenore Blake, Ron Blake, Brian Brock, Rebecca Bruyn, Craig Campbell, Hervé Canals, Nina Corwin, Mary Susan Convery, Cynthia Crowner, Laura Davis, Karen Frame, Seth Frohman, Charles Fuller, Ed Gebhart, Al Gentle, Mark Gianino, Ellen Greenhouse, Kay Gresham, Elias Guerrero, M. E. Hart, David Haughey, Ellen Highfield, Rafi Hoch, Jim Hopper, Brenda Ioris, John Jamieson, Nancy Janoson, Geneviève Joublin, Deborah Judd, Joel Kasow, Libby Keller, Burt Knopp, Colin Knox, Bob Lamm, Carol Lamm, Chuck Latovich, Rochelle Lefkowitz, Barbara Lerner, Hank Lerner, Injy Lew, Jason Lew, Janet Lewis, Wendy Maltz, Laura Markowitz, Kee McFarlane, Ricky McQuillan, Patrick Meyer, Marcie Mitler, Bernice Morgan, Robin Moulds, Bianca Cody Murphy, Randy Neff, Alexis Neophytides, Andreas Neophytides, Peggy Pahl, Nash Perkins, Michael Picucci, Stephen Powell, Phil Queeley, Peggy Rauch, Rose Rauch, Sol Rauch, John Reine, Avi Rose, Cindy

Rosenbaum, Kathy Samon, David Savitz, Stuart Simon, Ken Singer, Seymour Slive, Fred Small, Joan Sokoloff, Martin Sokoloff, Andrea Soler, Larry Spindel, Dan Stasi, Dan Sullivan, Lester Wall, Helene Wong, and Kathy Dee Zasloff.

I salute the young ones, lovingly parented, who give me hope for the future: Bette, Brendan, Brooke, Caitlin, Cassie, Claire, Danny, David, Eleanor, Eli, Eloise, Erik, Isabelle, Jackson, Jennifer, Jessica, Josh, JuJu, Justin, Katy, Kristen, Lizzy, Marisa, Max, Meghan, Olivia, Rachel, Robert, Ryan, Sean, Sophie, Toby, Veronica, and all the others.

I thank my parents, May and Gerson Lew, who continue to rise to the occasion, and the rest of my sprawling extended family.

Thanks to my neighbors on the Hill — Danny, Deborah, Emily, Gerry, Hank, Jim, Josh, Lynn, Martha, Mike, and Suzanne. You've created a *shtetl* in a city.

Thanks to all the past and present members of the "Soup Group," for years of wisdom and support.

My deepest appreciation to all whose experiences and insights are contained in these pages. You make the book sing.

Certain individuals were essential to the realization of *Leaping upon the Mountains*. They deserve special mention and heartfelt thanks:

— Oprah Winfrey, for starting this amazing process back in 1987.
— Zoya Slive, Richard Hoffman, Thom Harrigan, and Andrea Simon, for reading the manuscript in its many incarnations and providing valuable suggestions liberally seasoned with loving encouragement.
— Steve Klarer, John Hallum, and Dan (the Man) Zupan, for hours of help and patience with my cyber-fumbling, and Jim Sullivan, my gracious cyber-host.
— Felix Kramer, Norman Laurila and Ken Matticks, for contributing to "Team Leaping" in varied, wondrous ways, and the Team's foreign members, especially Chris Dawson (Australia), Alastair Hilton (England), and Mario Bourgeois (Canada).

— Richard Grossinger, of North Atlantic Books, for your help in negotiating the strange world of publishing.

— Michael Mendelsohn, for your talent and skill in designing the cover.

— Michael Woyton, desktop publisher extraordinaire, for combining technical competence, support, and unfailing good humor.

— Paul Nagano, for your generosity and the transcendent beauty of your art.

— Richard Hoffman — your words speak for themselves, so do your actions. You continue to challenge and inspire me.

— Thom Harrigan, my partner in all of this, through thick and especially thin.

— And my beloved Cosima — you comfort me when I'm down and don't take me too seriously.

I apologize to anyone I may have inadvertently omitted from this list. All of you make my life rich and full. You are responsible for the success of this book; its shortcomings are my responsibility alone.

"Leaping upon the mountains, skipping upon the hills...
...For, lo, the winter is past,
The rain is over and gone;
The flowers appear on the earth;
The time of singing is come,
And the voice of the turtle is heard in our land;
The fig-tree putteth forth her green figs,
And the vines in blossom give forth their fragrance."

— from The Song of Songs 2:8,10–13

Dedication

Fay Honey Knopp
(1918–1995)

In October of 1988, the first national conference on male sexual abuse was held in Minneapolis, Minnesota. It was a groundbreaking event in many ways, not the least of which was that attention was paid, perhaps for the first time at a major professional gathering, to *nonoffending male survivors*.

There are a number of reasons why I found the Minneapolis event personally meaningful. On the second day of the conference, I received from the publisher the first copies of my book *Victims No Longer*. I'll never forget being called to the hotel's front desk, tearing open a package, seeing the book for the first time, starting to cry and having two conference participants — women I didn't know — offer me hugs. At this gathering, I began to see how male survivors and counselors who work with them had been starving for a book that directly addressed their experiences. And I got my first hint of the degree to which my life would be affected by this book. It's hard to believe that this was less than a dozen years ago.

Among the many important speakers in Minneapolis that weekend was Fay Honey Knopp. Although I didn't know it at the time, Honey was to become my friend, mentor, and personal hero. Honey Knopp was the founder and guiding spirit of the Safer Society Program and Press. She was a longtime social worker, researcher, prison reformer, Quaker — and a Force of Nature. I hadn't known of Honey before that weekend, but as I watched her reach out to people, I began to fall in love. And I was reminded that support and encouragement remain the most valuable gifts we can give one another in this difficult and often isolating world.

Honey delivered the wrap-up speech at the end of the conference. Short and stocky, looking very grandmotherly with her white hair tied in a bun — and very rural Vermont in her turtleneck sweater, down vest, and long earrings — she took full command of the podium along with the hearts and minds of the audience. She said, "I'm a change agent." She continued, "I advise you all to get gray. It took me seventy years to look like this, and now I can get away with murder." (From what I have heard of Honey's work in prisons, that wasn't much of an exaggeration.) She proceeded to appreciate everyone who had anything to do with the conference, by name and what they had done. She spoke eloquently of the history of the survivor movement, its connection with other liberation and recovery struggles, how far we have come, where we are now, and the work we still have do. She didn't pull any punches; she was smart, tough, loving, and political. Her speech and her presence filled the room, and folks departed with renewed energy and dedication.

I kept in contact with Honey after we left Minneapolis. I had the pleasure of visiting a number of times at her home (and Safer Society's office) in rural Shoreham, Vermont. Honey and her wonderful husband, Burt, a beekeeper (no kidding), lived and worked in a large log house that offered rest and sanctuary to many people. For their fiftieth wedding anniversary, they bought themselves a canoe and paddled on the river near their house at the end of the workday.

As she did with so many others, Honey delighted in me and my work, supported me through hard times, and celebrated triumphs. She respected my skills and abilities far more than I did, and helped me believe in myself when I had the greatest doubts. Honey demanded the best of herself, and identified the best in others. Humanity in its many forms delighted her. Cruelty and inhumanity enraged her; she would not tolerate them. She inspired us to be our absolute best.

I particularly want to acknowledge what we have gained from Honey, because we have also lost her. Fay Honey Knopp died of ovarian cancer in August, 1995, a few days before her seventy-seventh birthday. She had worked hard to complete her last book. (It was published in 1996: *A Primer on the Complexities of Traumatic Memories of Childhood Sexual Abuse: A Psychobiological Approach* by Fay Honey Knopp and Anna Rose Benson, Brandon, VT: Safer Society Press.) I was told that, on her last night on Earth, she continued to focus her waning strength on the progress of the book. To the end, heavily medicated and struggling for breath, she remained fully alive to the ills and needs of society. I know it's the way she chose to finish her life — working passionately for justice and understanding.

Honey had been with her adult children through serious illnesses. She supported me (and many others) during a time of severe illness in my family. But she was not as ready to accept reciprocal help. In the last communication I received from her after her cancer diagnosis, she wrote, "Not to worry! Feeling fine — It's just one more challenge to a 76-year-old. No need to call — Just be happy and love life!"

Honey's memorial service, in mid-September 1995, was testimony to that love. People came to Vermont from as far as Arizona, and from all parts of her life. Memories of this extraordinary woman were shared by family, friends, and neighbors. People of all races and religions came — priests and ex-prisoners, antiwar activists and prison abolitionists, survivors and dairy farmers, old and young. Tributes were offered by famous people and ordinary folks, all speaking achingly of how Honey had touched and changed their lives. Honey's memorial was a powerful piece of history. I felt privileged to be there. But Honey's life message was not about words; it was always about *action* for humanity. As someone said during the memorial service, "When the memorial ends, the service begins." I know that the memorial that Honey most wanted was for all of us to commit our lives to fighting the loving fight — or, as some have called it, "Embracing the Journey." No one did that better than Honey.

What I hold in my heart of Honey Knopp is that she committed her life to reaching for the essential humanity in each person she met. Nothing was more important to her, and she let nothing stand in her way.

When we attempt to live as lovingly as possible, we won't always get it right. When we begin to transform jealousy into admiration and appreciation, we sometimes falter. But when we give up having to be perfect and instead commit ourselves to taking responsibility for our mistakes, learning from them, and rededicating ourselves to doing what is most human, we are accepting Honey's vision of a healthy world.

I dedicate this book to Honey Knopp — her vision, the difference she made to the world, and the inspiration she continues to provide. Honey, you touched so many of us. We miss you and will honor your life by embracing the journey.

Foreword

by Richard Hoffman
Survivor and author of *Half the House: A Memoir*

"Freedom is the right not to lie," Albert Camus once wrote, and in this book, brave men assert that right and exercise that freedom in the service of healing one another. Their truth-telling is the untelling of many lies and distortions about boyhood and maleness, about the sexual abuse of boys, and about recovery.

Here are the voices of men who have seen through many lies, suffered to bring their exiled spirits home, and struggled to regain their freedom. Here you will find a brotherhood that does not rely on adherence to doctrine, girding for war, or subjugation of others. Here you will find new men.

You will find no cheap locker-room advice here. No counsel to "get over it," "shake it off," "suck it up." You will find no pernicious talk about the "necessity" to forgive. Nor are you likely to encounter any psycho-babble about "the cycle of violence," so-called "false-memories," or "the profile of the (sic) male sex-abuse victim." These are the voices of men — white, black, Asian, Hispanic, straight, gay, bisexual — regarding themselves honestly and confiding to us what they see and understand.

Many of us who will read these pages have suffered the trauma of boyhood sexual abuse, and we will be strengthened and inspired by the generosity and honesty we find here. Before any of us can commit to the hard work of recovery, we have to believe that it's real, that it's possible to find a way out of shame and confusion, and that there is a kind of power (besides power over those who are weaker) worth claiming. There is abundant proof positive in this book.

These powerful words of witness challenge the stereotype (which exists to shame victims into silence) of the forever wounded, the psychologically damaged, the emotionally crippled. But it would be a terrible waste if these words were not also heard by those who are fortunate enough not to have undergone such suffering. Telling the truth and listening to it are the reciprocal processes by which we build and maintain a vital community. No one has the right to stay ignorant of atrocity.

Listening gives people the occasion and the reason to find language to speak the truth. It encourages the teller to find the right word, not the expected one; not the acceptable word, but the one that truly corresponds to experience. Listening restores faith, integrity, authenticity, freedom.

Mike Lew is a consummate listener. To those who know his work — his writing, his speaking, his workshops, his steadfast advocacy, this book is a much anticipated blessing. He has modeled for all of us that quality that invites the truth to emerge in all its subtlety and complexity. He has brought together a moving chorus of men's voices here. Arresting as each one is, taken together they demonstrate what those of us who know Mike have heard him say often: "Because the sexual abuse of children takes place in secret, in isolation, recovery must take place in the open, with others."

More and more men are coming forward, empowered by their brothers (many of whom have allowed themselves to be instructed by courageous sisters). They are propelled by the knowledge that standard-issue male consciousness is inadequate to anything but displacement of their pain, and can only exist in the context of abusive hierarchical power. For men, rejecting the shame and silence that are the usual legacy of sexual child abuse involves defection from a bankrupt ideology that defines power as dominion, supremacy, command.

According to Czech dissident writer Ivan Klima, "The dreams of the powerless are either to flee to safety or to gain power." Looking back at my own life, it seems to me that its entire course, until recently, could have been plotted using those two coordinates.

I fled my hometown, scene of my shame. I fled the working-class background that marked me for sneers and dismissals. I fled the church that further shamed me. I fled my self, whom I was taught to see as a loser. I looked for safety in muscular strength, weight lifting myself into an armored pose. I looked for safety in women's arms. I looked for safety in the bottle's anesthesia.

The alternative dream, of wielding the same kind of power I had suffered under, was abhorrent to me. Stuck, I settled for a life in which time passed, meant little, and accrued to nothing.

Only when I'd understood that there was another kind of power — not abusive power, not power over other people, but the power to speak the truth — could I admit that the dream of safety is part of the problem. To feel the kind of safety the first dream promised would require me to betray what I knew just as surely as the second dream, the dream of power, would require me to deny the pain of my boyhood. Both dreams are one and the same: the first says, "Now I can never be hurt again"; the second shrugs, "Better you than me." Both are as sterile and solitary as dreams must be.

When you speak the truth, you wake from this terrible delusion. At first there is pain, like the blood returning to a numb limb when we've slept too long, too drunkenly, too deeply. You wake to a world where others are suffering from the onslaughts of abusive power: where children are still being violated, women are still being raped, men are still being beaten, and where shame still drives the deadly machinery of disempowerment and disintegration. But it is also a world where, once you commit yourself to the struggle for wholeness, recovery, and justice, there is joy and laughter, solidarity and strength — a world of truth telling and compassionate listening, as evidenced by the book you hold in your hands.

Richard Hoffman
Cambridge, Massachusetts

Introduction

Boston, Massachusetts

When I undertook this project, I didn't want to write another *Victims No Longer* — that book had already been written. It was time to take my work to the next step, looking at where we've come in male recovery in the 1990s — at what is now possible that wasn't before. I wanted a book that would encourage people during the early stages of their recovery, and provide acknowledgment and perspective to those who have been at it for longer.

I finally wrote a book proposal and was met with unanticipated resistance. Even though *Victims No Longer* has sold well over 130,000 copies, and sales continue steadily more than ten years after its initial publication, I was told that the market was saturated and there was no need for another book on male survivor issues. The proposal was turned down by my publisher and many other publishing houses. My literary agent suggested, "...they...feel that the men's market is too narrow. ... If you are still interested in the project, it may be time to explore self-publishing." It was the same old discouraging song I had heard years ago about *Victims No Longer* and about men's issues, in general. It meant that I wouldn't receive an advance that would allow me to take time off to write, and I wouldn't have a deadline. Historically, I haven't been very good about setting my own deadlines — I'm too easily distracted.

But survivors, therapists, and friends kept asking when my next book was coming out. They kept urging me to write more. I knew that those publishers were wrong — the need and interest were still out there.

Although the process slowed for a while, ultimately my stubbornness got me going. I decided that this book had to be written, and (like the Little Red Hen of children's literature) if I wasn't going to get any help from the publishing establishment, I would do it by myself. Unlike that famous fowl, however, I have received lots of support and encouragement from friends, colleagues, and the recovery communities. I decided to take it on, risking my time, energy, and savings. I would trust my own judgment and the urgings of people I respect, and go against conventional "wisdom." I think the results prove us right. Here goes.

THE GOAL OF *LEAPING UPON THE MOUNTAINS*

During the past decade, a great deal has been written about recovery — recovery in general, sexual abuse recovery, and even male survivor issues. Treatment programs have been developed, insights shared, theories promulgated, clinical modalities explored — and entire schools of thought have been established. As in many fields, certain theories and practices have come to be so widely accepted that they have taken on the aura of TRUTH. When fact is assumed, it is easy not to bother checking to see whether it makes practical sense.

I'm not a researcher. I have never attempted to quantify the components of recovery — and I am not going to try to do so now. My goal is simple — to write a book that FEATURES male survivors and will BE USEFUL to survivors and their allies.

Over the years, I have had ample opportunity to witness male survivors engaged in a visible process of change — courageously, persistently, and (ultimately) triumphantly. I've noticed that some things have worked for my clients, and others haven't. In general, approaches that have worked best are those discovered or modified by the individual himself — resources that speak to that person's needs at a specific point in his recovery.

Many survivors, desperate to "do it right," have tried to learn what they "should be doing" to recover. When a person's need is urgent, and his level of self-doubt is high, he is likely to be vulnerable to any quick fix or "authoritative" suggestion, regardless of whether it works for him. Survivors and their experiences are widely diverse; one size can never fit everyone. People have different needs at different points in their recovery. The recovery process is rarely clear-cut and is never simple or linear. Therefore it is essential that survivors find the specific support, activities, information, and treatment strategies that make the most sense to them — and be open to changing these strategies in response to their evolving needs.

Despite great diversity within the survivor community, there is commonality. Reinventing the wheel is a colossal waste of time; we can benefit from one another's experience. If you are a survivor, it is possible that someone else has discovered something that you will find useful.

We know that every individual's recovery needs to proceed at a reasonable pace and level of intensity. There is nothing to be gained and a great deal to be lost by attempting to hurry a process that requires its own time. As I have said elsewhere, faster and more intense are not necessarily better. Attempting to force your pace most likely will lead to disappointment, self-doubt, self-criticism, and even retraumatization. Before adopting any particular suggestion about recovery strategies, it is a good idea to examine your own personality, needs, and preferences. No matter how good an article of clothing may look on someone else, if it is the wrong size, style, or color for you, it won't fit. Of course you can try it on, but try not to be discouraged if it's not a good fit; there are many other possibilities. This is true of therapies and therapists, books and courses, workshops and programs, philosophies and religious practices, and all sorts of other activities. Keep on trying until you discover or develop the ones that work best for you.

In figuring out what works for you, you can avail yourself of the experience of others who have explored similar territory. There is a lot of information available. When you go to a library or video store, you don't come home with every book or tape. You may have read reviews that interest you. You might get recommendations from friends whose opinions you value. You peruse the shelves, find a few titles that seem interesting, and take home one or two to try out. You then find that some don't make sense, don't fit your interests, are too simple or too complex, or just don't speak to your mood at the moment. So you return some uncompleted, are indifferent to others, enjoy parts of some others — and a few you want to read or view again and again. Occasionally something that doesn't have meaning at one period of your life may become important later on. And we all have experienced outgrowing some interests and values as the circumstances of our lives change. I invite you to remain open to new possibilities (and to revisiting old ones), employing this openness when you explore suggestions from other male survivors. Remember, these are possibilities, not requirements. Nothing is mandatory except treating yourself with respect and caring.

In the literature about "treatment" of survivors of sexual child abuse, I have yet to see any real investigation of *what survivors themselves identify as most important to their recovery*. I always learn best by going to the experts, and — since we now have a reservoir of experience with recovery — there are lots of experts out there. You are probably one. Some years ago, I began asking the experts (male survivors) what they have found most useful at different points in their recovery.

I've always been wary of suggesting specific recovery techniques, either to professionals who work with survivors or to groups of survivors. The reason for my reluctance is that when a new technique is mentioned — especially by a so-called expert — it can be received as "gospel." Rather than seeing it as one possibility to be explored (and perhaps rejected), it may be taken as a requirement of healing. When this happens, some professionals try to use the technique with all their clients whether or not it makes sense to do so. [In a 1965 movie called *The Cincinnati Kid*, Ann-Margret plays Melba, the wife of a small-time gambler called Shooter (Karl Malden). In one scene, Melba is sitting on the floor assembling a jigsaw puzzle, using a manicure set to trim some of the puzzle pieces. Shooter asks her, "Melba, why do you do that?" She replies, "So it fits, stupid." As she continues to tailor a piece with her nail file and clipper, Shooter says, " You'll ruin the puzzle. Now, that doesn't go in there." Pushing the reshaped piece into the puzzle, Melba replies, "It does now."] While it might be possible to force some recovery techniques into place, if they don't fit your needs, they will not contribute to a coherent picture. Survivors who jump uncritically into a new recovery fad can find themselves disappointed when it isn't relevant to their situation. This lack of "fit" isn't a problem if they are able to test it and discard it as inappropriate. But if their self-esteem is too fragile, they may wrongly interpret its lack of success as further evidence of their own failure.

When I began asking male survivors about resources they have discovered or developed over the years, I was not attempting to develop a universal theory or treatment program. It wasn't even formal, systematic research. In part, I was checking whether assumptions that I (and many of my colleagues) had been making were congruent with the experience of men in their own recovery. I figured that the more options are made available, the greater the chance that an individual will find something personally useful; more and more people would learn that opportunities for healing are abundant.

How I Went about It

I began the project very informally, without a long-range plan. At male survivor workshops, I posted large sheets of paper bearing the heading RESOURCES THAT I HAVE FOUND HELPFUL. Throughout the course of these workshops I invited participants to share specific resources that they have employed to further their recovery. Other workshop participants could then look at the list, try anything that seemed like a good idea, and ignore what didn't feel right for them. An additional benefit of the list turned out to be that some survivors discovered that things they had taken for granted were, in fact, important healing strategies. They learned that it isn't only psychotherapy and twelve-step programs that contribute to recovery; everyone has a great deal of experience and information to share. Here are two examples of those lists, generated during weekend workshops. The contributions were anonymous and are presented here exactly as they were listed, without explanation. When a specific resource was listed more than once, I included the repetition.

Here is the first list:

Taking Care of Me by Mary Kay Mueller

Journaling

Tai chi

Journaling

"There's a Hero inside You" by Mariah Carey

Talking

Volunteer work with survivors and parents/guardians of

Seeing/hearing former Miss America, Marilyn Van Derbur speak

Drawing (Cra-Pas are GREAT!!)

Abuse Web sites

Transcendental meditation

EMDR therapy — eye movement desensitization and reprocessing

Groff breathing

Psychodrama

Art therapy

Drama of the Gifted Child by Alice Miller

Hobbies

The twelve steps (of AA)

Friends

Love relationship

Psychodrama

Friends

Working on the grounds/rocks/dirt

Survivors of Incest Anonymous (twelve steps)

Journaling and drawing

Amusement parks

Renee Fredrickson audiotapes on (1) relationships and (2) career (for survivors of abuse) located in Minneapolis

The Celestine Prophecy by James Redfield

VOICES in Action conferences (<u>V</u>ictims <u>O</u>f <u>I</u>ncest <u>C</u>an <u>E</u>merge <u>S</u>urvivors)

A lot of open, loving, vulnerable people

Forgiveness

Being here

This is the second list from a different workshop:

Running/exercise

Water

Creating Sanctuary by Sandra Bloom, M.D.

Trauma and Recovery by Judith Lewis Herman

The Artist's Way by Julia Cameron

Victims No Longer by Mike Lew

The Holy Bible

Psychotherapy

Bathing

VOICES in Action annual conferences

The Seat of the Soul by Gary Zukav

Talking about it with others

Vipasanna meditation retreats in Shelburne Falls, MA

The Transcended Child by Lilian Rubin

Resilient Adults by Gina O'Connell Higgins

Anything by J. D. Salinger

The Psalms. In particular, check out Psalm 18 or 21

Telling Secrets by Frederick Beuchner

No should'ing

Gordon Lightfoot album *Salute* poetically describes a recovery process.

Raising a Son, the book

Raising a son, mine

MASSF (Male Abuse Survivors Support Forum) at http://www.noahgrey.com/massf

12-step recovery from sex and love addiction

Group therapy

Prayer

Self-care

Letters to a Young Poet by Rilke

Survivors of Incest Anonymous (SIA) 410-282-3400

Pema Chodron, books and tapes (Buddhist meditation)

The Linkup at www.thelinkup.com (clergy abuse)

Songs: "Don't Give Up" by Peter Gabriel

"What about Now" by Robbie Robertson

"Don't Cry" by Seal

The Healing Game album by Van Morrison

Movies: *The Boys of St. Vincent* and *Sleepers*

Those are just two of many such lists created by workshop participants. Over time, I noticed that certain themes kept repeating. Others, no less important, seem to be more idiosyncratic — helpful to a few people, relevant to a particular life experience or a specific point in a person's healing. One reason I haven't included exact statistics is that numbers aren't as important as the way resources speak to you. When you find your soul mate, your true love, or your passion, it doesn't matter that the rest of the world doesn't feel the same. When you discover a career or activity you love, you don't need everyone to enjoy it equally. Similarly, if only one person suggests a resource that strikes a responsive chord, then it is "the right one." It is relevance and fit that make a difference, not consensus. On the other hand, I decided to let you know which responses were more or less frequent, assuming that something that has worked for lots of other male survivors may have a good chance of proving useful to you.

If nothing else, I felt it was valuable to get people thinking about what *works for them* — letting them see (regardless of how it may feel) that their recovery hasn't been a random affair. We all have made significant discoveries and choices in leading and changing our lives.

I've been extremely fortunate. *Victims No Longer* provided me with contacts beyond my wildest dreams. Since its publication, I have had the incredible opportunity to do workshops and trainings and speak at conferences in many parts of the United States and Canada, as well as Europe and Australia — experiences that allowed me to meet and speak with thousands of male survivors, their partners, families, and friends, female survivors, therapists, and other professionals. I've been in communication with survivors and professionals in every state or province in the United States, Canada, and Australia, as well as people in Argentina, Austria, Belgium, Brazil, Cayman Islands, Canary Islands, Colombia, Costa Rica, Czech Republic, Denmark, Dominican Republic, Egypt, England, Finland, France, Germany, Greece, Guam, Haiti, Hong Kong, India, Ireland, Israel, Italy, Japan, Jordan, Kenya, Malaysia, Mariana Islands, Mexico, Netherlands, New Zealand, Nigeria, Norway, Palau, Pakistan, Peru, Philippines, Poland, Puerto Rico, Samoa, Scotland, South Africa, Spain, Sweden, Switzerland, Trinidad, Turkey, Ukraine, Wales, and Zimbabwe. I've listened to what these folks had to say and I've learned from all of them. A great deal of what is contained in this book is the result of years of listening to these experts. Some — those who replied to my questionnaire — are quoted directly. Others are incorporated less directly, threads in a tapestry of recovery.

THE REQUEST FOR RESOURCES

The piece of *Victims No Longer* that evoked the strongest reader response was the personal statements by male survivors. When I thought about writing a second book, I knew that I wanted a significant component to be men directly sharing their successful recovery experiences. After years of hard work, we have plenty of these experiences to call upon. I wrote up a very simple, nonscientific questionnaire and began to distribute it in a very simple, nonscientific way. I gave it to everyone I encountered. I sent copies to survivors and professionals on my mailing list (in every U.S. state and Canadian province, and other countries whenever possible). I displayed stacks of them at male survivor workshops, conferences, and professional trainings. I sent batches to survivor organizations such as VOICES, ISTI, and Linkup. Every time I received a letter, phone call, or request for information, my reply included (unless clearly inappropriate) copies of the questionnaire and release form. I asked colleagues to help me with this project, and utilized several people's computer expertise to post the request on various Web sites.

It was neither a random sample nor statistically valid. Like many survivors beginning their exploration of recovery, I employed whatever resources I could find. I used whatever was at hand and enlisted the help of anyone around. I am grateful to all the individuals and organizations who took time to respond.

Here is a sample of one of my request forms:

To: **MALE SURVIVORS OF SEXUAL CHILD ABUSE**
From: **MIKE LEW**

REQUEST FOR RESOURCES

Male survivors display extraordinary creativity and resourcefulness in finding and developing resources for healing. I believe it is essential that these resources be shared. A major focus of my next book will be male survivors' experiences of what has been of significant value to them in their recovery. This is a request for you to respond to any or all of the following four statements, as specifically as possible, in a sentence or two. Please type or print legibly:

1. An important resource(s) during the *early* part of my recovery was...

2. As my recovery progressed, I found help and encouragement from...

3. In support of my recovery *today*, I focus on...

4. Something I would like to say to other male survivors is...

Contributions that are selected for publication may be included as a whole or edited. Contributors will be identified by a first name (of their selection), age, and state or province. To be considered for publication, contributors must sign the attached release. Thank you for your help.

◆ ◆ ◆ ◆ ◆

A sample of the release form follows:

RELEASE

Mike Lew has my full permission to quote, in whole or in part, my response to his request for resources for his next book. I understand that if my contribution is selected for inclusion, I will be identified only by a first name of my choosing, my age, and state or province, and that I shall receive no payment for my contribution.

I wish to be identified as (First name only)

_____

My age is _____

State/Province _____

Full name (Please print)

_____

Address_____

_____

Signature_____

Date _____

Please send this release, with your contribution attached, to Mike Lew at The Next Step, P.O. Box 1146, Jamaica Plain, MA 02130, USA

The Responses

I distributed thousands of these questionnaires in no systematic fashion, and received hundreds of excellent responses from male survivors in every state of the United States and the District of Columbia, all ten Canadian provinces, as well as forty-four other countries. They came from men of diverse backgrounds, races, religions, ethnicities, linguistic groups, sexual orientations, educational and economic levels, ages, and life experiences. They have different abuse histories and are at various places in their recovery. There are fathers and those abused by their fathers, clergy and survivors of clergy abuse — all types of men, all manner of experience. They range in age from nineteen to seventy-five, with the greatest number in their thirties and forties.

The responses are as diverse as the men themselves. Some themes are repeated by many, others offered by only one or two individuals. Some were expected; others are surprises. All are interesting, and I hope you find them helpful. I have included as many as possible, usually with exact quotes from the contributors. At times I have added my own comments. Some contributions have been edited in order to maintain focus on the most powerful aspects of the response. Wherever there has been editing for brevity or clarity, I have attempted to preserve the tone of the writer. Any failure to do so reflects my limitations, not those of the contributors.

I have tried to include as many different voices as possible, but was unable to include every response. I don't pretend that what is presented here is completely representative of male survivors worldwide. There is an overwhelming imbalance of replies from the United States and Canada. A disproportionate number of entries are from the states and provinces where I know more people or where men have greater access to recovery resources. There may be certain regions, cultures, ethnicities, or classes where men have greater freedom to talk about abuse. Whenever I received only one or two responses from an area, I used every bit that was relevant, but I don't know how representative they are. If a writer responded with only a word or two, I only included it if it was different from other contributions. It is likely that writers who are not native English speakers would communicate more fluidly in their own language — and a few had to depend upon another person to translate for them. Even with these obstacles, I think the quotes provide a clear and consistent picture of the reality of recovery.

Although I asked people to respond to my questions in a sentence or two, many chose to do otherwise. Some individuals expressed their frustration with a format that limited them to a few sentences, and several came up with elegant solutions. For example, in his accompanying letter, **Gordon, 45, British Columbia, Canada,** wrote,

> " When I was getting ready to answer your four questions, my wife asked if I had read the part that said answer in a sentence or two. I went immediately into shock.... I cannot pin down a specific resource for a specific time frame. I did have something to say to other male survivors. My problem was the part about in a sentence or two. I reached back into the past for a solution...my son's (high school) English teacher assured us he was the next Shakespeare. Many of my son's sentences were the length of a short story if not a short novel. So I would like to give you a sentence that I feel explains my recovery journey to other male survivors."

He proceeded to write an eighteen-line sentence (which is included in the answers to Question 4), concluding with the following:

> "Well there it is in only one sentence. I feel an English teacher might have something to say about the lack of punctuation and too many 'ands.' "

Paddy, 49, Queensland, Australia, wrote,

> "I have received your letter 'Request for Resources' and this puts me in a quandary as it is very difficult to address this issue in so few words. I have decided to compromise by acceding to your format and also to provide a context in which what I say will make more sense beyond the few word statements."

Some folks expressed displeasure at the lack of specificity of my questions. I understand that many survivors have a hard time with lack of structure, but I consciously chose nonspecific questions to encourage writers to express themselves as freely as possible. I think the results speak for themselves.

It pleases me that quite a few men ignored my suggested restrictions or got around them in creative ways. Some took several paragraphs or even pages to reply; others responded in a word or two. And still others offered their contributions in the form of essays, poetry, fiction, or personal history. You will find examples of these creative solutions throughout the book.

Some contributions weren't direct replies to the questionnaire. Here and there, with permission, I used pieces of creativity that were originally presented at workshops and trainings. I am not a literary critic, but I believe that each one speaks from the heart and has special meaning for men in recovery.

This *haiku* was written and read by **Bill, 51, Washington, D.C.,** during one of the weekend male survivors' workshops we hold each summer at the Kirkridge Retreat Center in the Pocono Mountains of Pennsylvania. Its simplicity and purity first led me to include poetry in this book.

An Experience at Kirkridge

Perched on mountain side

Demons exposed, dance in light

Our paths continue

Many contributors expressed appreciation for the opportunity to share their experiences, and speak to other survivors. **John, 43, Wales,** wrote,

**"I am delighted to have the opportunity to contribute....
Thanks again for the chance to speak."**

Michael, 40, New Jersey, asked me to consider including his poem. I'm more than pleased to be able to do so. In a few words, he offers understanding, appreciation, encouragement — and a call to action.

The Mighty, The Weak, The Meek

by One of the Many

Here we stand,
   afraid of what we thought were the mighty.
Ashamed of what we had become, huddled secretly
   amongst our thoughts.

Heads held down for so long,
   backs weak against the task.
How we came to be thus,
   the questions we ask!

Come my child, be whole again,
   in ways you know not how!

Humbly go and tell your tale,
   carry yours and share the pain
      with all the ears that can hear!

Buckle not to the rage!
   On our backs,
      we the meek,
         carry the new age!

It is I who must thank John, Michael, and all the others. How generous of them to help me and then thank me for it. I'm certain, as you read their words, that you will add your appreciation to mine.

Several men noted that writing their answers was, in itself, a useful recovery exercise. For example, **Ram, 50, Manitoba, Canada,** wrote,

> **"It took me a while to digest that this might be used in your book and caused me to reflect on all the steps and stages I had experienced in this process."**

It was another example of how to help oneself by helping others.

While all the communications I received are important, not all were appropriate for this book, and therefore not every response is included. There were moving stories of childhood trauma and ongoing effects of sexual child abuse. There were responses from men who are just beginning the recovery process. Their stories — in all their pain, fear, anger, and grief — need to be told, but that is the subject of another book.

Leaping upon the Mountains is not about the effects of abuse. Much has been written about that subject — in *Victims No Longer* and elsewhere. Therefore, I haven't included responses that focus on the abuse, and have edited parts that are oriented in that direction. Those responses are no less important; it is necessary that survivors talk about the abuse — over and over — for as long as they need to. It is essential that survivors are listened to, believed, and supported through their painful recounting. But this book is about the successes. It is recovery-focused, and the responses that are included reflect this orientation. While never denying the pain and difficulty of recovery, these messages provided by so many male survivors — in so many ways — confirm what I have always maintained to be the truth: *Recovery is possible, it is real, and it matters!* The quotes in this book speak to that reality far more eloquently and persuasively than I ever could.

This is not a work of fiction. It is a compilation of many truths — of many realities. It is a quilt, pieced together from many men's stories. The picture they form offers an impressively triumphant pattern.

MESSAGES OF ENCOURAGEMENT

During trainings and workshops, I often refer to the degree that our lives are bombarded with messages of negativity and discouragement. We are told that life is bleak and hopeless. I call these words and images "death messages." Although such messages are found everywhere, they are neither helpful nor accurate.

I believe that, as therapists, survivors, allies, or simply caring humans, it is essential to contradict destructive ideas; we must search for messages that reflect the reality of human strength, caring, resilience, courage, creativity, and love. I'm not suggesting denial; we cannot ignore grim realities of life. But there is far more to human existence than unhappiness. The world is richly beautiful, infinitely diverse — and so are we. The contributions to this book reflect that wealth, beauty, and diversity. And there is much more available to us than I was able to include. Whenever we find life-affirming resources, in any form, we must support them, acclaim them, and share them with clients, friends, and loved ones. We must tend our gardens and value every flower. When we discover a quote, song, story, painting, poem, film, artist, performer, novel, dance company, or activity that reminds us of the reasons to be alive and human, we must embrace it and let others in on it.

For every despairing, hopeless, nihilistic musician, there is another who is honest, loving, and human. Some are well known; others take some discovering. We must find song writers and musicians like Nancy Day, Fred Small, Bill McKinley, Mariah Carey, Stephen Sondheim, and The Flirtations who speak out specifically and forcefully about abuse and recovery. (See the Resource Section for information about obtaining recordings by these artists.)

Scott, 41, Michigan, wrote,

> **"Thanks for the tip to witness the joy and healing nature of Nancy Day. Her music is almost as powerful as her presence."**

We must also discover (and rediscover) those — like Pete Seeger, Sweet Honey in the Rock, Tuck and Patti, Donovan, Ravi Shankar, Bob Marley, and many others — who show us beauty and strength that transcend pain. We need to listen to music that engages the soul and lifts the spirit. Whether it's pop, rock, folk, gospel, jazz, reggae, classical, world music, new age, or whatever, we must find songs (as Stevie Wonder put it) in "the key of life."

Fred Small is a wonderful singer and songwriter who lives in the Boston area. A number of his songs, including "Everything Possible" and "Light in the Hall," have profound meaning for survivors. He has generously given permission to reprint the lyrics to "I Will Stand Fast." Fred's words are those of a committed ally. The world will be a safer place when all victimized children and adult survivors are believed, understood, and supported this effectively — when all allies display his degree of confidence in recovery. In his songbook, *Promises Worth Keeping*, Fred introduces "I Will Stand Fast" with these words:

> **"All of us get hurt. It helps if there is someone who will listen gently to our story, hearing us out without judgment or criticism, giving us room to feel our feelings without interjecting their own. I am grateful to know that this song has been widely used to assist the healing of sur-**

vivors of child abuse. But whatever our history, it has not always been easy. We all need someone who will stand fast for us, as we in turn will stand fast for them."

I Will Stand Fast

The echoes of childhood whisper violence
Cold wind beating out of the past
Rage in your throat muffled silence
Hold on I will stand fast

In the darkness your guardians had left you
Cold wind beating out of the past
None to hear your cries none to defend you
Hold on I will stand fast

CHORUS:
I will stand fast I will stand fast
You are safe in the daylight at last
Nightmare and fear they have no power here
I will stand fast

I will listen to the terrors that tried you
Cold wind beating out of the past
I will cradle the child that breathes inside you
Hold on I will stand fast

Though you take the shape of a hundred ancient
    horrors
Cold wind beating out of the past
Though you strike at me and flee into your sorrow
Hold on I will stand fast

CHORUS

Birds flash upon a branch in winter
Cold wind beating out of the past
Ice in the sun begins to splinter
Hold on I will stand fast

You will walk with no fetters to bind you
Cold wind beating out of the past

**All the love you have wanted will find you
Hold on I will stand fast**

CHORUS

Words and music by Fred Small
Copyright 1988 Pine Barrens Music (BMI)

We need to read and reread books and poetry that remind us of the value of the human heart and the human soul. We must return to the special books of our childhood (like *The Little Prince* by Antoine de Saint-Exupéry) and rediscover why they spoke to us. We must discover gems like *The Crock of Gold* by James Stephens to experience the pleasures of embracing life in all its diversity and the glories of human language. If we find a contemporary novel like Barbara Kingsolver's *The Bean Trees* (where love and human ingenuity triumph over abuse), we must let it be known. There are many survivors (like Maya Angelou and Richard Hoffman) who have learned to thrive and who have made significant contributions to this literature of life.

We need to be with people who share our commitment to life. All of us have spent far too much time around discouraging, hurtful people. It's time we let go of negative attachments and make room for health and joy. Truly, the best is yet to come.

Every time we discover someone or something that makes a difference, we need to acknowledge it, support it, and share it. We can't assume that everyone has equal knowledge of resources or access to them. If you find a poem like Mary Oliver's "The Journey" or Denise Levertov's "Living Alone (III)," share the wealth. Display your discoveries prominently. Pass them on.

It was suggested to me that I repeat here a story that I included in *Victims No Longer* — about the time I suggested to a survivor that there is a huge range of territory between the extremes of black and white. He replied, "Oh, you mean shades of gray." I answered, "Yes, but also red, blue, green, orange, and magenta." We owe it to ourselves and others to experience and share every manifestation of beauty and creativity.

Survivors and their allies are reclaiming all that was taken away from them. A few years ago, at the national conference of V.O.I.C.E.S. in Action (the national organization of incest survivors), Mary Rizzuto was at the podium delivering her presidential address. She stood proudly, dressed in red and black. There are some who would have avoided wearing that combination of colors, which is often associated with satanic rituals, fearing that they would trigger flashbacks for survivors of cult abuse. But I saw something quite different; Mary was making a statement that we are taking back *all* the colors. Survivors are ready to reclaim the true meaning of words and concepts that have been perverted. Red and black are just colors, and rituals are wonderful ways to mark important events in the human life cycle. We are creating healthy, joyous rituals and celebratory ceremonies; no longer will abusers be permitted to co-opt and destroy the good things of life.

I continue to learn from my contact with survivors. In what follows I hope to display proudly some of what I have gleaned from these experts on healing. You will have an opportunity to experience the diversity, intelligence, and creativity of male survivors. I offer this book to you as a celebration of their successful recovery — and yours.

UNEXPECTED ENCOURAGEMENT

Over the years I have learned that people are capable of being abundantly supportive and generous. Although I have met my share of individuals whose pain has translated into anger and destructiveness, I continue to be encouraged by many more who haven't allowed past injuries to destroy their goodness and humanity. Time and again, when I have felt overwhelmed and discouraged, people have given me new hope and energy. Some of these boosts have been subtle (someone not even knowing that he or she is making a difference), but they are enormously important to me. I hope this book helps to express my appreciation to all my allies — especially those I neglected to thank adequately at the time.

Never undervalue the effect you can have on others. Sometimes a small, inadvertent act makes all the difference. One well-placed

appreciation, thoughtful gesture, small recognition, slight encouragement, or personal connection — can produce unexpected ripples.
I'll give you several examples:

In attempting to elicit the widest possible range of response,
especially from places where I had few contacts, I sent a follow-up
letter with a second Request for Resources. I had some qualms
about doing this, not wanting to exert pressure on survivors who
weren't ready or were uninterested in responding. I didn't want anyone to feel guilty about not contributing, or let their sense of
responsibility and obedience to authority overcome self-care. I just
didn't want to nag.

In the midst of all of my second-guessing and self-criticism, I
received a response form accompanied by a letter from a male survivor. It contained a splendid "reframe" that eased my concern. **Bill,
38, Alaska,** wrote:

> **"Thank you for your second letter asking for input to your
> second book. Your first letter stimulated a desire to con-
> tribute, though inertia — and many aspects of my abused
> past — delayed my writing. I appreciate you caring
> enough to send a second letter. Enclosed are the answers
> to your questions, the release form, and copies of some
> poems I wrote to help grieve the loss of my mother (who
> sexually abused me for many years).**
>
> **"I first bought your book in 1990. I 'lost' it for sev-
> eral years. I bought a second copy two years ago. I have
> yet to read it. I believe some of the reasons include a fear
> of opening the subject alone...and my conditioning that a
> man can not be abused. The last part is the hardest for
> me. I logically know the abuse happened when I was
> child, yet as a 5'11", 188-lb. man, my feeling is I should
> have been able to stop any abuse. So it goes; my recovery
> continues.**
>
> **"Even though I have yet to read your book, I thank
> you from the essence of my soul for writing it, and writ-
> ing a second book. Just knowing that someone cares
> enough to write about this subject, to give me a book to
> point to (and) say, 'Yes, men are incested by their moth-
> ers,' is part of a powerful step in my healing. Just typing**

> these lines brings tears of joy, and healing.... With warmth
> and nourishment, Bill"

I still haven't met Bill, but his generosity of spirit represents one of many ways I have learned and grown from the insights of male survivors. It reminds me that if you don't get what you need the first time, it's OK to try again.

It was good, too, to be told that some people found the exercise of answering my questions useful. In accompanying letters, **Oliver, 53, Massachusetts,** wrote,

> "Thanks for this opportunity. It's been helpful for me to respond. (I've cried just while writing the little I have, and it's OK, I've still got work to do)."

and **Bob, 65, Delaware,** said,

> "Reading the set of four questions served to reactivate some of the pathways to recovery that had been gestating."

Although it wasn't my reason for asking these questions, I'm pleased that it had that result for Bob. Taking stock can be very useful.

I met **William, 46, Arizona,** briefly, at a conference where he was facing a frightening encounter. A passing suggestion — one that I've made many times to countless people — made a difference to him. In the letter accompanying his response, he wrote,

> "Thanks so much for your reminder to keep breathing! I would also like to take this opportunity to say thanks for your words of encouragement when you witnessed me falling apart in proximity of the bishops. You simply reminded me, 'You can do this, William.' Sometimes I forget what I am capable of doing. Those few words will stay with me for a long time."

In fact, I hadn't known that William was "falling apart." I saw someone who seemed to be having a hard time, and a little encouragement never hurts. I'm glad I was able to help; I'm grateful to William and all the others who took time to let me know it. I encourage you not to assume that people are aware of their importance to you. Tell them! Be specific as to how they have made a difference. It will be good for both of you. And please, when people tell you you've helped them, don't let embarrassment or modesty make you deflect their appreciation. It doesn't matter that you think "it was nothing." It was important to them; you made a difference in someone's life.

In his letter, **John, 58, Washington, D.C.,** echoed William's comment. He wrote,

> **"I shall never forget the tool of: 'breathe.' I forget I can use it all the time, but then I take a breath, and it comes back."**

It's an important thing to remind people — and it's easy, too. Whenever you notice someone holding his or her breath, you can smile and suggest, "Breathe." Chances are you'll get a responding smile or laugh. And be sure to keep reminding yourself. Remember that breathing has two parts. These are:

1: IN.
2: OUT.

For best results, both parts must be included. Otherwise you will turn very blue.

I thank you all. I thank those who have contributed their experiences and insights to this book; I thank those of you who did not. If you respected your own needs, privacy, and boundaries by deciding not to contribute, that, too, is an important piece of healing and self-care. Good for you! Don't waste any time beating yourself up about it. Continue to take the best possible care of yourself.

A REMINDER TO THE READER

I have a request before you go on with this book. PLEASE resist the temptation to measure yourself against the men who contributed their experiences in these pages. No good comes of worrying about whether you are at the right place in the recovery process, or why someone else seems to be ahead of you. You are exactly where you should be. You couldn't have begun your healing a minute sooner than you did. Don't fall victim to old messages that undermine your self-confidence. The information included in this book is intended to be helpful, not discouraging. The more you resist the impulse to beat yourself up, the more you will recognize that you have already made brilliant progress in locating resources for yourself and creating a uniquely effective pattern of recovery. Other male survivors have resources to offer you — and you have much to offer them. Give yourself a break!

Part One

EARLY RECOVERY

The data included in the following sections are from individuals with whom, directly or indirectly, I have some connection. Many are people I haven't met — some have written to me, attended a lecture, or asked to be on my mailing list. Some received copies of the questionnaire from friends, family, or helping professionals, and others have responded to requests posted in various locations on the Internet. I don't know where some responses came from. However, it is likely that each person is acquainted with me and/or *Victims No Longer,* and that acquaintance must have influenced some of their answers. But the information they provide is theirs. *Leaping upon the Mountains* is intended to *feature* survivors and be *useful* to survivors. I hope you are able to use any part of it that makes good human sense to you.

The first question asked male survivors to respond to the following statement, as specifically as possible, in a sentence or two:

An important resource(s) during the *early* part of my recovery was...

I did not try to define early recovery, allowing each individual to decide for himself. The responses may reflect differences in how people perceive the stages of their own recovery.

What follows presents the responses by general category. There are other ways the answers could have been organized, as there is a good deal of overlap (and occasional ambiguity). To make the material easier to handle, I created categories that seemed reasonable to me. If they don't make sense to you, feel free to tinker with them.

Unless otherwise indicated, quotes from the contributing male survivors are indented and in boldface. And except where indicated, they are from survivors living in the United States.

BOOKS AND READING

By far the largest category mentioned in early recovery, consisted of *books, reading*, and other forms of *taking in information*. It is not surprising that so many survivors begin their active recovery by reading whatever is available. It is the safest and most confidential way to seek information. The reader has complete control over the pace and location of his work, and some control over its intensity. Before a survivor is ready to take action — or even talk about the abuse — reading can show him what resources are available and the level of public understanding of his issues. It lets him experience his feelings about the situation and think about his next steps.

During early recovery, responses in this major area focus on *obtaining information* and *understanding*.

> **"In early recovery I was really scared of other people, particularly of other survivors. Literature then was so helpful and 'safe'!** *Victims No Longer* **spoke to me in a way that was nurturing, gentle, and most of all 'SAFE'! I saw how others had gone before me and how they had done it. I took what I liked and shelved the rest." — Larry, 32, New York**

> **"...it enabled me to understand myself and why I'm so isolated and afraid." — Gordon, 57, New South Wales, Australia**

Fully half the responses mention *reading in general* and *learning* about survivor, abuse, and recovery issues.

> **"Always books have been a refuge...to escape into a beautiful world...kept me alive." — Stefan, 51, South Africa**

> **"Bibliotherapy. I read many books, as much as I could find, on sexual abuse and recovery, in general. At the time, there were very few books specifically written by and for men. While this was a hindrance in that reading of 'women's pain' and identifying with it lent to my shame, I have long since come to realize that sexual abuse is not about sexuality and that any survivor, male or female, will be similarly affected." — John, 32, Newfoundland, Canada**

> "As I read, I gathered bits of information which seemed to make sense or jog a memory for me." — Doug, 35, California

Many cite *specific books*, often for specific reasons.

> "...books on sexual child abuse. When I first began to acknowledge my abuse, I wasn't ready to 'talk,' but I needed nonjudgmental information. (I) could get that from books. My biggest challenge was trying to read books, by and about women, which always dealt with male abusers. That was a struggle. It felt like the books were indicting me by association. I would start and stop, out of frustration, many times trying to find some relevant information. Finally I found *Victims No Longer*, one of the first books — if not the first — that spoke to male survivors about male sexual child abuse. My recovery started to expand exponentially once I had that resource. It spoke to me about my processes, my feelings, and my patterns. It opened the door for me to really accept that this happens to little boys. Once I could accept that, it was easier to accept that my abuse started when I was four years old. This book helped me take my next step, which was to seek out support groups." — Paul, 34, Washington, D.C.

The above quote is typical of the many men who write of the importance of reading information and personal statements that speak of specific experiences of *male* child victims and adult *male* survivors, experiences that mirror their own.

> "...written TO men, not about men. It was suddenly OK to be a victim, to cry, to have female perpetrators." — Benn, 32, Georgia

> "...the relief of recognition..." — Alford, 55, Michigan

> "What a wonderful feeling it was...to see mirrored before me and come to light what I was living inside. There it was! At last, someone was talking about male survivors of sexual child abuse and the effects it has made in a man's life!" — Daniel, 39, New Brunswick and Ontario, Canada

Since these are responses to my questionnaire, it is not surprising that *Victims No Longer* is cited so many times. For many men, connection to other male survivors broke through their isolation and established empathy — often for the first time.

> **"I discovered it by accident and it was a startling revelation."** — **David, 61, Michigan**
>
> **"...Victims No Longer. Several of us 'very scared' survivors would get together and read and release."** — **John, 38, Oklahoma**
>
> **"...it was like Androcles taking the thorn out of the lion's paw."** — **Scott, 43, Brazil**
>
> **"...it let me know that I was not alone in my struggling to make sense of the world, that I was not alone in my personal suffering, that others had lived the same tortures! I read 'my story' in that book and some initial healing took place in my tears of sadness over their hurts."** — **Mark, 34, West Virginia**
>
> **"After breaking a twenty-five-year silence, it was very reassuring to know I was not alone...or crazy."** — **Brad, 35, British Columbia, Canada**

The two other books cited a number of times are *The Courage to Heal* by Ellen Bass and Laura Davis and Alice Miller's *Thou Shalt Not Be Aware*.

> **"While it was written for women, *The Courage to Heal* offered a path to understanding my situation. It led to your book, which later brought me to communication with other male survivors. It was my beginning."** — **Ramesh, 40, India**
>
> **"Alice Miller fought against the medical bullies."** — **Jürgen, 36, Germany**

Several men write more generally about the importance of *reading other men's stories, education about male survivors,* or *formal education.*

> **"When I began to learn that how 'broken' I was feeling was not a matter of being odd or different or strange, but rather a matter of what had happened to me, the world opened up. To read that other people were feeling what I was feeling — and not feeling what I was not feeling —**

and to know there was a place to look forward to in my future." — Jim, 26, Massachusetts

"Reading other men's stories gave me some hope of eventually recovering." — Jon, 47, Minnesota

"Reading about male survivors, commonalities we share. Reassurance I was not alone in my horrible experience of physical and emotional pain. Men are allowed to feel pain and cry!" — Ron, 52, Missouri

"An important resource during the *early* part of my recovery was my college studies in psychology. It was in the study of behavior that I first started to understand that it was not my fault for the abuse and that I could not have done anything to prevent it." — David, 35, Wyoming

Nineteen other books are each mentioned once. (They are no less important to the men who listed them.) These include nonfiction and fiction, recovery, abuse, men's issues, and other themes. As with any of the suggested resources in this book, you are encouraged to investigate those that appear interesting to you and ignore the rest. See for yourself — and please don't limit your exploration to this list. If you find something that is helpful or meaningful, I invite you to share it with me and with others. Please add your own discoveries to the list. There are lots of resources out there. I'm not aware of all of them, and we can use them all.

The other books cited in response to Question 1 are listed here alphabetically by author:

Soul on Ice by Eldridge Cleaver
Absent Fathers, Lost Sons by Guy Corneau
The Right to Innocence by Beverly Engel
The Wounded Male by Steven Farmer
Repressed Memories by Renee Fredrickson
Catching Fire by Merle Fossum (audiocassette)
Outgrowing the Pain by Eliana Gil
Something Happened by Joseph Heller
Abused Boys by Mic Hunter
Primal Therapy by Arthur Janov
The Flying Boy by John H. Lee

Taking a Chance on God by John J. McNeill
The Drama of the Gifted Child, For Your Own Good, and
    Breaking Down the Walls of Silence, by Alice Miller
The Wounded Healer by Henri J.M. Nouwen
The Road Less Traveled by M. Scott Peck
Male Survivors by Timothy Sanders
The Dreamworks Manual by Strephon Williams

Specific reference information about these and other works cited by male survivors can be found in the Resource Bibliography at the end of this book. Please remember that I am not recommending these books, just compiling a list.

> **"...books written by other survivors...in particular I drew much comfort and strength from Timothy Sanders and Laura Davis. The early days were the most difficult for me because I did not remember anything...and then I began to get only snatches of uninvited memories. This was most distressing. Reading the experiences of others helped me through this time; I learned that I was not alone at the very time when I felt most alone." — John, 43, County Mid Glamorgan, Wales**

> **"...books...which made it clear that abuse could happen and not just be dismissed as an Oedipal fantasy." — Doug, 46, New York**

> **"...books opened up a conduit to lost feeling." — Paddy, 49, Queensland, Australia**

Some men write about using their computers, the *Internet* and the *World Wide Web* (www) during early recovery. I suspect that, as this vast resource becomes more widely available, we will see more and more survivors begin their recovery by gleaning information and connecting with others via the Internet. In this unprecedented way, they can maintain their anonymity as long as they need to, while reaching out of isolation. Over the past year or two, there has been a great increase in the number of Internet resources available to survivors.

> **"...the forum on CompuServe called the Human Sexuality Forum. In that forum is a section called 'I Was Abused' (IWA), which is limited to people who have experienced**

some kind of abuse (sexual, physical, or emotional) in their lives. When I first joined the forum, I thought almost no other men had been sexually abused like I was, but I found that many others had indeed experienced sexual abuse. IWA was the first place where I told anyone that I had been sexually abused, and I received a lot of support from the members of the section. I was able to disclose my past in IWA because I felt safe in the anonymous atmosphere of the on-line community. It was also in IWA where a person referred me to a resource that was helpful to me as my recovery progressed, SIA (Survivors of Incest Anonymous)." — Doug, 33, California

"...the M.A.L.E. Web page at http://www.male survivor.org/ which gave my first real information on male survivors, the resources available, and where to find them." — Warren, 31, Ontario, Canada

Other sources of information cited (one mention each) are *television*, *radio*, and unspecified *newsletters*.

"...various John Bradshaw PBS [Public Broadcasting System] specials..." — Pete, 30, California

"...hearing Susan Forward on a talk radio show...speaking of the behavior of incest (at the time) victims. I cried because, in her descriptions, I thought she had mentioned my name." — Peter, 37, Massachusetts

Finding clear, accurate information, however it is obtained, has been essential to a great many recovering survivors. But it is important to remember that the fact that something is in print does not guarantee either its accuracy or its usefulness. Use your best judgment to determine what makes the most sense for you.

SAFE ENVIRONMENTS

It is necessary to find or create safe settings for active recovery work. As might be expected, many more people mention the primary importance of a *safe environment* during the early part of their recovery than later on. Although it is difficult for any environment to *feel* safe to a survivor (particularly when he is taking those first, tentative steps out of isolation), it is absolutely essential that there be some space that *is* safe. How can it be possible to begin the difficult, painful work of recovery when one is in danger and needs to be constantly vigilant? Later on, when the individual has established greater equilibrium — when he has a surer sense of his own successful survival — physical environment becomes less significant. This probably explains why about twice as many people mention a safe place in early recovery as in mid-recovery, and about six times as many as in later stages.

During this early part of recovery, the most commonly cited safe places are *treatment settings*. References are made to *hospitals, residential treatment centers*, and *alcohol* or other *drug rehabilitation*.

> **"No way I could do what I had to do and still lead my every day life. I had to get away to a place where I could get treatment." — Terry, 49, Tennessee**

> **"...where I discovered what was done to me was incest and it was not just [ML — !] physical violence. There was a reason — a name — for this insanity in my head." — Aaron, 29, New Mexico**

> **"I never fully faced my abuse until...in an alcohol rehab treatment center. Earlier, I had felt that I handled it because I broke away from my perpetrator and kept him at bay with anger and hatred. In reality, I hadn't faced it, grieved over it, or brought it into true focus. Other cases of similar abuse in my group therapy gave me the courage to discuss it openly." — John, 61, Maryland**

It is clear that, for many survivors, *sobriety* is necessary for starting their recovery. When addictive behaviors are understood as reactions to abusive experiences (whether in an attempt to numb the pain, as a reflection of negative self-worth, or as some other form of survival strategy), giving up the addiction represents commitment to life, health, and growth.

> **"...to stop hiding behind booze and the fourteen-to-sixteen-hour workdays." — Jim, 58, Kansas**

> **"I cleaned out my head and went about my work." — Les, 60, New Zealand**

> "Once I acknowledged I was a drunkard, I looked at everything with a clearer eye." — Magnus, 37, Sweden

A few responses refer to a *safe place* without indicating the specific components of safety.

> "...a place where I could relax..." — Clay, 24, Oregon

> "...somewhere safe from them. To stop running." — Jose, 41, Argentina

As you will see later, the type of physical environment that is important to these men changes as they progress. None of the information is startling. What comes as a surprise is that, given how many survivors have attempted "geographical cures," relatively few individuals include physical environment in their responses. Only about 6 percent cite this category in response to the first question, and even fewer to the second (3 percent) and third (1 percent).

> "I had to leave my village.... First to Istanbul where I would be 'invisible.' Later, traveling for help to England and America." — Kemal, 48, Turkey

PROFESSIONAL RESOURCES IN EARLY RECOVERY

INDIVIDUAL COUNSELING

Many men write of the value of *individual counseling* or *therapy* during early stages of recovery. While therapy continues to be an important resource throughout the recovery process, the nature, focus, and emphasis shift in the answers to the three questions. Fully a third of the returned questionnaires make some reference to individual counseling or therapy in response to Question 1.

> "For me, individual counselling was essential. It provided a safe, supportive, and challenging environment in which to reconnect with my pain and begin the process of sharing it for the first time. I had managed to block out a considerable amount of the details and a host of addictions and self-abusive behaviours kept the pain equally distanced. Reconnecting with that require professional guidance and support. I also believe today that a male

counsellor made a difference. While I have since had female and male therapists (and benefitted from both), the fact that the first one was male facilitated a lot of trust and healing. I had lived my life up to that point being afraid of men with the assumption that the only way that I could win approval or safety was via alcohol or sex. Developing trust in a male counsellor, and having that trust held sacred, enabled me to avail of other support such as A.A. [Alcoholics Anonymous]. Eventually, I was able to trust other men with my 'shame-filled secrets' and have them accept me and share with me and support me. Recovery has often felt like a process of 'reconnecting' with my gender." — John, 32, Newfoundland, Canada

"...a therapist who wasn't afraid of my pain and could respond to it on an emotional level. I was describing one of my first memories to her early in the process of recovery. I spoke in the flat monotone, the dissociated voice so many survivors use in describing the pain inflicted on them. When I finished and looked up, I saw a tear run down her cheek. That was an incredible opening for me. It was then OK for me to feel how bad it felt." — Olin, 42, Vermont

"I didn't know anyone who could help me. I sought professional counselling." — Julian, 30, Hong Kong

Adding individuals who list some form of *group therapy* brings the therapy numbers up to 42 percent. (This figure does not include peer organizations, programs, meetings, workshops, conferences, seminars, and retreats. They will be discussed later.)

At this early point in recovery, far greater importance is given to making a therapeutic connection with another individual than with the activity itself. Three times as many survivors mention their *individual therapist* or *counselor* as cite the process of individual counseling/psychotherapy.

"...finding a doctor who HEARD and knew...She saved my ass. Not only did she listen, she HEARD. She was THERE." — Benn, 32, Georgia

"...working one-on-one with a therapist, then joining a survivors' group he leads." — David, 54, Colorado

> **"...a lucky and indispensable find — a good therapist...in Prague."** — Douglas, 45, Czech Republic

> **"I saw Dr._____ weekly at first...sometimes more frequently. It was most valuable."** — Sam, 31, Nigeria

Responses suggest that this emphasis changes dramatically as recovery progresses. There may be any number of explanations for the shift. One possibility is that, early in recovery, the survivor may still be looking for a "savior" — someone who will magically make things all better.

> **"The violence in my childhood began in infancy. During...years of individual therapy I was acting as a naive helpless child. I placed my 'self' in the therapist's hands. I placed all my troubles in their in-baskets in the unspoken belief that they would perform their curative magic and someday hand me their formulations and my whole self. My use of confession as a Catholic was a precursor for this model of therapy as well."** — John, 58, Massachusetts

> **"I found my guardian angel who took the form of a psychologist."** — Hector, 58, Mexico

It may be that finding a safe individual, committed to establishing and maintaining good boundaries, provides the necessary contradiction to prior experiences. Again, we see that regular, healthy contact with another human being offers a way out of isolation.

> **"It was hard to believe that this woman wouldn't violate me like my mother. But she never did."** — Val, 30, Florida

> **"I thought he would disappear. I expected that he would give up and leave me, but he remained week after week, month after month until I began to trust him."** — Mohammed, 42, Pakistan

The *therapist's commitment* to the survivors' recovery, *belief* in his worth and the value of the process, and possession of *specific information and resources* about recovery are all precious gifts.

> **"He was behind me every step of the way."** — Joel, 34, Connecticut

> *"...my therapist who reminded me of what an incredibly resourceful and creative person I actually was."* — William, 46, Arizona

> *"...my therapist taught me that I was important..."* — Keith, 31, Quebec, Canada

> *"...told to me many times over, if I would not give up, my life would improve."* — Klaus, 56, Switzerland

> *"...answered my questions...showed me where to look for more..."* — Luis, 22, Costa Rica

> *"...a therapist who knew what he was doing."* — Tom, 61, Maine

Commitment to *ongoing work together* is, for some, the first evidence that someone can actually listen, believe, and tolerate their revelations of abuse.

> *"...to trust my therapist with the facts about what happened."* — Roger, 44, Florida

> "He would not abandon me. How could I abandon myself?" — Juan, 67, Spain

VALUABLE THERAPEUTIC QUALITIES

At all stages of recovery, men address the importance of finding a counselor who embodies particular qualities, professional and human. Certain words keep appearing as male survivors write of therapists who helped them break through their fears, fostered trust, and made a significant difference to them.

> "It could not have been easy. I was cold, angry, and suspicious. Her warm understanding melted my walls." — Ali, 53, Egypt

> "Meeting a therapist who I could learn how to trust." — Charles, 45, Illinois

> "Never before had I met such a man." — Thomas, 45, Germany

> "The process was so different from anything I had experienced. My therapist loved me, held my hand, taught me to cry and laugh and understand that it was not my fault."
> — Dale, 42, Hawaii

The quality mentioned most frequently is PATIENCE.

> "...a great, patient therapist. It goes (in my situation) very, very, very slow." — Todd, 32, New York

> "...my therapist, who was patient with me, especially when I was the most impatient with myself." — Rod, 48, Rhode Island

Good therapists understand that a survivor must be in charge of his recovery. This is confirmed again and again, as men detail the importance of working with counselors who allow them to move at their own pace, neither pushing for greater intensity nor attempting to slow the process.

> "...a therapist who had the patience to allow me to wend my own way, even though it was clear I didn't know where the fuck I was going or what I was doing in his office." — Bob, 65, Delaware

> "I had need to proceed slowly, slowly, slowly. My fear was large. Never was he impatient with me." — Ryszard, 22, Poland

> "...having an understanding and patient therapist who let me go at my own pace and never pushed." — Dan, 28, Massachusetts

While accepting the responsibility to point out that working at an unhealthy or unrealistic level of intensity can result in retraumatization, therapists must not attempt to slow things down because of their own fear. On the other hand, it is essential that therapists do not — out of impatience or frustration — force a pace that isn't healthy for their clients.

Other attributes that keep appearing in descriptions of valued therapists are SUPPORTIVE, GENTLE, KNOWLEDGEABLE, VALIDATING, and GOOD LISTENER.

> *"...a knowledgeable, gentle therapist who constantly and consistently encouraged me to expand my other resources..."* — Tom, 40, Michigan

> *"My therapist provided support and expert information."* — Peter, 43, South Africa

While only a few definitions of the valued traits are offered, it is clear that the writers know exactly what they mean by them — and how to recognize them.

> *"I couldn't have told you what I was looking for in a counselor — but I knew when I found the right one."* — Pat, 42, Nebraska

Many other words and phrases are used; some are variations of previously mentioned themes. Taken together, the answers provide an excellent picture of what survivors value in a therapist, counselor — or any other ally.

> *"...a knowledgeable, caring, and supportive therapist that stood by my side as I journeyed through the painful memories and gave me guidance on dealing with them..."* — Curt, 43, Wisconsin

> *"She would stand with me (not for me) while I did the work myself."* — Thor, 55, Washington State

Traits that are valued by survivors in their therapists include *encouraging, consistent, skilled, trusting, trustworthy, nonshaming, nonjudgmental, working on their own issues, accepting, genuine listening, no advice, caring, providing information and guidance, safe, challenging, experienced, sympathetic, understanding, kind, empathic, comfortable with emotions,* and *real.* Listen to their voices:

> *"...kept right on telling me that I could do it until I said 'Hey, maybe he's right!'"* — Van, 41, Colorado

> *"...always kind to me, always hopeful..."* — Carlos, 47, Peru

> *"...well trained...in detecting the symptoms of abuse and using skills to extract this from within me."* — Jeff, 43, Nova Scotia, Canada

"...a skilled, patient and trusting therapist..." — Jim, 55, Michigan

"...a counselor you can trust to help face and accept the painful stuff and get past it...the next step!!" — Pete, 49, New York

"...said I should be proud of myself. The shame is theirs." — J.V., 28, Kenya

"...my nonshaming and nonjudgmental therapist, who was the first person to listen to my account of childhood and teenage abuse and exploitation without discounting and minimizing my experience..." — Michael, 30, Ohio

"...she had been working hard on her own issues. I credit her with saving my life." — Nick, 47, Texas

"...let me speak the truth..." — Teishiro, 34, Japan

"...a therapist who was very accepting of me and genuinely *listened* to me *without* 'giving advice' or suggesting answers to my horrible nightmares. He validated me as a person." — George, 61, Washington State

"I felt like Sally Field. I wanted to shout, 'You care! You really care!'" — Matt, 20, Iowa

"...showed me how to locate the information and support I had been searching for." — Tony, 44, Nevada

" ...kept bringing me back to the topic — he didn't let me get away with diversions." — Arthur, 65, Oregon

"...the sympathetic and understanding ear of my abuse councillor, she was easy to talk to and listened to what I had to say through tears and offered assistance in referrals to other avenues of self-help." — Christopher, 33, Victoria, Australia

"...kindness, real kindness. Not just another patient. Not just another job." — Ray, 34, Idaho

"...she helped me verbalize my fears and anger..." — Dan, 34, Ontario, Canada

> **"...down to earth. No bullshit. No therapizing." — David, 27, Oregon**

It is interesting that none of these terms describes a particular therapeutic theory or counseling practice. One again, the qualities of the "singer" are more important than the particular "song." That is why survivors have been able to make stunning progress working with good counselors using all sorts of therapies. There are human qualities that can't be taught. Just as the ability and humanity of a good therapist will probably shine through regardless of what type of therapy is used, a bad therapist will not be redeemed by a particular clinical modality.

Whatever the reasons, it is clear that *healthy human connection* is essential to recovery. As I have observed many times, abuse happens in isolation; recovery occurs in the company of others. Many male survivors have found the courage to contradict cultural messages that stereotype "real men" as tough, stoic, silent loners. Those types aren't real people — they are more like cardboard cutouts. Real men feel. Real men make contact.

> **"I refused to allow my returning trauma to isolate me from the support I needed." — Bob, 43, California**

> **"...to find someone to talk to..." — Ismail, 40, Malaysia**

Human connections are as vital in the early stages of recovery — when the survivor is breaking through secrecy and silence to reach out for information and resources — as later — when he is solidifying and consolidating his gains and effecting lasting life change. Although the focus shifts, necessity for healthy interaction remains. We need one another. We cannot afford to be isolated again. Never again!

> **"I could not go back into hiding ever, so I had to become visible." — Wim, 28, Netherlands**

Within the categories of *individual therapy* or *counseling* and *therapist* or *counselor*, most of the responses are nonspecific, although a few individuals mention a specific form of therapy (e.g., hypnotherapy) or therapist (e.g., couples counselor). After reading the first draft of this manuscript, one of my colleagues expressed surprise that although so many people refer to their spouses and partners, there is no mention of family therapy and very little acknowledgment of couples counseling. It was an interesting observation, and I spoke of it to another reader, a male survivor. He suggested that survivors are very proprietary about their recovery, and may not view their couples work or family therapy — however important — as part of their *individual* recovery. I am curious to hear what others think about this.

Also a bit surprising (given the current popularity of antidepressants) is that only a couple of men indicate that they benefited from *medication*. The types mentioned are antidepressants and antianxiety prescriptions.

> **"I was suicidal...and had not yet identified childhood sexual abuse as a significant issue...anti-anxiety drugs...at least kept me in limbo until true healing could begin." — John, 49, Massachusetts**

GROUP THERAPY

The form of *group* therapy most frequently cited as helpful during early recovery is the *male survivors' group*.

> **"Being in a group with other men who were also survivors of sexual abuse was crucial to my healing. Group shatters one's denial about what happened and helps you to truly realize the seriousness of the abuse and its effect on your life." — Sean, 29, Massachusetts**

> **"I can honestly say that my therapy recovery began...when I entered my first treatment group for male survivors of sexual and violent abuse during childhood.... In less than two months of beginning to share with other male survivors, many things became obvious. I had never identified myself with another human being in my life. I had identified with authors and fictional characters. I had never wanted to be a member of any group of people as soon as I had gotten to know them and 'seen through' them. For the first time in my life, I did not feel superior to others in the group and wanted to 'fit in' with them rather than stand out and stay above them." — John, 58, Massachusetts**

> "I could not possibly have been able to speak of my fears of women, talk about what happened to me and the effect it had on my life, in the presence of women." — Chris, 57, Ohio

> "...weekly attendance at a male survivors' group led by a psychologist. I 'lucked' into this group just as my first memories and realizations surfaced...and have done a large part of my healing within this supportive and safe group of men." — Kristian, 52, Saskatchewan, Canada

> "...my feeling of warmth and acceptance from my male survivors' group." — Alford, 55, Minnesota

Describing his recovery group in "The New Frontiersmen," **Alford, 55, Minnesota,** offers us a powerful, poetic appreciation of his fellow male survivors.

> **The New Frontiersmen**
> **1**
> We are the new frontiersmen,
> Strong like our forefathers,
> Scouting a darker landscape
> Than those who have gone before us.
> Male survivors of sexual abuse,
> Made hesitant by the past,
> We meet together weekly
> To share forbidden history.
> Men of sixty, men of thirty years,
> We know no generation
> But that of fellowship.
> Straight men, gay men,
> Seeking a single stronghold.
> Different in aspect, united by our pain,
> We have answered a call,
> A summons to be healed.
> **2**
> Cognizant of our commonality,
> Alive to our own uniqueness,
> Our mentor leads us gently—
> Each to his own rhythm,

Each in his own time—,
A trip into the interior,
A trek into the soul,
The inner frontier,
Determined to free the men children within us.

3

Brave men. Strong men,
Daring to be open with each other,
Casting off the burden of shame.
Awkward in our first attempts
At breaking silence
(Like raw recruits brought newly to the field),
Using each other as sentinels.
Men who forge weapons from words,
From reenactments of childhood memories.
Men united against a common enemy,
Naming aloud our sexual abusers,
And in doing so,
Laying to rest unquiet nights
And days of shadow.

4

Certain in our cause,
Certain in our safety together,
We learn each other's boundaries.
We touch each other's souls
—a healing bear-hug, a hand upon a shoulder—
It is enough.
Men together—vulnerable, beautiful,
Learning to cry openly,
Eager to become our own wound dressers.
Working toward our well-earned freedom,
We will face the future on our own.
But for now we travel together—
One in purpose, one in kinship.

5

We are the male guardians of the future.
Storytellers who have learned to share our passage
From trial to victory.
We are the new frontiersmen.
We will tell our sons to tell their sons
And make the world a safer place for men children.

In early recovery, male survivor groups are listed as frequently as all other types of therapy groups combined. However, we will see that the importance of group therapy increases sharply later in the recovery process. Other types of therapy groups mentioned (in descending order of frequency) are *general issues groups* (or unspecified group therapy), *survivors' groups* (gender not specified), and *men's groups* (unspecified focus).

> **"My group let me know that I didn't have to face the demons alone." — Bo, 56, Nebraska**

> **"I never trusted men. I didn't want to be a man. My men's group showed me that men aren't all abusive." — Randy, 36, Tennessee**

A number of other men mention *workshops* (e.g., a male survivors' weekend), *retreats, conferences* (e.g., V.O.I.C.E.S. in Action), and *educational seminars.*

> **"...going to workshops and meeting others who are dealing with the same issues that I am." — Jim, 42, New Hampshire**

> **"...a weekend retreat with other male survivors, and a week-and-a-half retreat with other men." — Rick, 35, North Carolina**

> **"...the weekend retreat for (male survivors) of sexual abuse at Kirkridge...was the true beginning of my journey of recovery." — Gug, 46, Pennsylvania**

> **"...absolutely nonthreatening approaches to this issue, i.e., *educational* seminars..., outpatient counseling (Short term, then run!!!), books on men's issues." — Tony, 32, South Dakota**

The following excerpt is from a letter written by **Tom, 44, Pennsylvania,** shortly after his first male survivors' workshop. It is representative of many men's reactions to the power of a shared recovery experience:

"...how much that weekend meant to me. It was the first time I was ever (knowingly) in the company of other men who had been sexually abused. Hearing some of their stories and talking with some of them had a tremendous effect on me. I finally got to see and hear that I'm not the only one who feels scared, anxious, and I'm not the only one who feels like a real 'fuck-up.' Finding out that we all share many of the same feelings and personality traits makes me somehow feel more normal than I did before last weekend.

"Since returning home...I find that I'm a little 'calmer' than I was before. I'm also starting to feel some anger about the abuse I experienced, and it feels great to finally have some anger!!!

"Friday night, and again on Saturday I wrote the name of my perpetrator on the large sheet of paper that you had hanging on the wall. I had never done anything like that before, and I found it sort of hard to do. At your suggestion, I also started referring to my perpetrator by his name, instead of calling him 'my pastor.' I discovered during the weekend (and still) that it helps bring on anger by calling him by his name. I shared that with my therapist yesterday — she then referred to him by name five or six times during our session and it really helped to piss me off (but also to finally focus my anger where it belongs)....

"I've been in touch with two other guys from the Kirkridge weekend, and it helps me to correspond with them. Later tonight, I'm planning to write to one or two more of them.... I want to say it again, being with other guys who grew up with experiences similar to mine was very, very helpful to me. Before that weekend, I really didn't know that there were other people who feel, act, and react the way I do. I'm also looking into joining a group of male survivors...who meet once a week. Groups always scared the hell out of me, but I think I'm ready now."

◆ ◆ ◆ ◆ ◆

Important as they are, these single events are less than half as significant during early recovery as later on. What seems hold up from early through mid-recovery (although not, as we will see, in later stages) is the importance of a category that includes *peer organizations, programs, meetings,* and *principles.*

> **"...the peer support group that let me share my emotions, pain, anger, and fears in a safe 'external' environment and to know that I wasn't alone as a male survivor." — Curt, 43, Wisconsin**

The largest number of responses in this category refer to *Alcoholics Anonymous* (AA).

> **"...AA. I had to become sober before I could begin to look at whatever was making me so angry and anxious. The honest, open, and willing approach suggested in dealing with my alcoholism was a powerful model in dealing with sexual and emotional abuse." — John, 58, Washington, D.C.**

> **"Alcoholics Anonymous was also a huge help in the 'early days'. Because (in 1984) male survivor groups were not available to me, AA became an important place for me spiritually. Taking a personal inventory of how my abuse had (emotionally) harmed others, was crucial to my recovery." — Jim, 35, Maine**

> **"...AA and the twelve steps — spiritual awakening." — Doug, 57, California**

The next most frequently mentioned organizations are *Survivors of Incest Anonymous* (SIA) or *Incest Survivors Anonymous* (ISA).

> **"SIA showed me that I didn't have to settle for being a victim." — Patrick, 42, Rhode Island**

These are followed by unspecified *twelve-step groups* or programs, *Adult Children of Alcoholics* (ACOA), *Adult Children Anonymous* (ACA), *Sex and Love Addicts Anonymous* (SLAA) or *Sex Addicts Anonymous* (SAA), unspecified *peer support groups*, and *phone lines* or *hotlines* (e.g., The National Recovery Hotline).

> **"...opening up and sharing my struggles with newfound twelve-step friends." — Rick, 35, Montana**

"...ACOA meetings. ISA was too intense and I had to begin to learn to feel before I could start delving into the deeper painful stuff." — Paul, 36, Pennsylvania

"I learned the differences between healthy and unhealthy behaviors by watching others. I experienced encourage-ment and validation as others listened to me and expressed agreement or disagreement with my observa-tions. I learned some of the 'body' lessons, which I had been numb from for many years...good touch and bad touch. I was searching for explanations. Many of my ear-liest realizations were very painful. The ACA group was a platform on which I could experiment." — Ed, 46, Michigan

Fifteen other groups receive a single mention each. They are *Al-Anon, V.O.I.C.E.S. in Action, Codependents Anonymous* (CodA), *Focus group* (Cult Awareness Network), *S.A.S.A.M.* (Texas), *MESA* (Scotland), *Reevaluation Counseling, Adult Children of Dysfunctional Families, Kempe Center* (Denver, Colorado), *Onset Program* (South Dakota), *Looking Up* (Maine), *Delawareans United to Prevent Child Abuse, Catholic Charities*, a *men's SIA group*, a *professional group* (unspecified), and an unspecified *social group*.

"I met several men in those meetings who shared their own childhood abuse histories. Their stories helped me to know that I was not alone." — David, 57, New Mexico

"...a support group to go to twice a week, called S.A.S.A.M., that Chad Butler started." — Dwayne, 44, Texas

"MESA...a support group for males who have been sexu-ally abused. People who listened to what I had to say." — Jim, 24, County Strathclyde, Scotland

"...the men's SIA support group. During the...years I attended, I received and gave a quality of support *not* possible in the *same way* in a mixed group." — Frederick, 54, Michigan

"In the early part of my recovery, I did a lot of crying. I was able to feel my sadness and sob in an Adult Children of Dysfunctional Families support group. I was more in touch with the sadness in this group of twenty or so people than alone with my therapist." — Mark, 30, Indiana

Statements like Mark's make it clear that there is often — at any stage of recovery — safety in numbers. Recognizing the importance of group support, we must oppose whatever denies access to that safety. We must take a stand against anything that would keep us separated from our allies. To help us understand how racism (and other forms of oppression) inhibit recovery, I asked M. E. Hart if he would write something that addresses recovery issues for male survivors of color. He generously contributed the following article.

A PERSON OF COLOR: OVERCOMING BARRIERS TO GROUP PARTICIPATION

by M. E. Hart, Attorney-at-Law

I am an African-American male whose sexual abuse, perpetrated by multiple abusers, began at age four and lasted for fifteen years. The camaraderie and understanding of the support groups I worked with over a three-year period helped me rebuild my self-esteem and regain control of my life.

During my recovery, however, I noticed a troubling trend. I was, in most cases, the only African-American in the groups I attended. Other African-Americans would not stay in the groups for more than three or four meetings. In response, I immediately began reaching out to persons of color when they would first come to a meeting. I tried to be supportive and encourage each to continue in the program. In most cases, I was not successful.

As a former Legal Advisor to the Director of the Office of Human Rights in Washington, D.C., and an avid student of civil rights, I have spent well over ten years studying and specializing in discrimination and race relations as it applies to employment and other opportunities for people of color. When I began group work, in 1987, to advance my recovery process, I was initially surprised at the extent that race affected that process as well.

In professional settings, I could objectively evaluate cultural differences and keep my emotions separate—or so my legal training led me to believe. But when issues of race intimately affected my recovery process, I could not move forward until I put those issues in their historical perspective in relation to the events in my life.

From my experiences, and in discussions with other African, Latin, or Caribbean survivors, I have identified barriers that persons of color may have to overcome to reap the full benefits of group participation in the recovery process. These barriers may arise through having to face *our* own *external* and *internal* prejudices.

EXTERNAL PREJUDICES

The most difficult external prejudice we face is a dysfunction of our larger society—racial prejudice. This problem was readily reflected in a 1990 survey of the University of Chicago's National Opinion Research Center, which found that:

> "Fifty-three percent of nonblacks believe that African-Americans are less intelligent than whites; 51 percent believe they are less patriotic; 56 percent believe they are more violence prone; 62 percent believe they are more likely to 'prefer to live off welfare' and less likely to 'prefer to be self-supporting.'"

This is a snapshot of the psychological environment people of color face every day and have faced for generations. So, from life experience, we must expect that any group we attend will have at least some people who may share these beliefs. It is easy to understand how this social reality can act as a barrier to honest communication in mixed-race meetings, especially when the subject is a very intimate one.

I can honestly admit that it is difficult to speak of personal issues when you feel you will be perceived as "less intelligent" and "more violence prone" than other members of the group—especially when the group is dealing with the violent crimes of sexual abuse. Claudia Black, Ph.D.,

M.S.W., writes about this dynamic in her book *Double Duty*. She explains:

> "Many people of color learn at a very young age that their color is not okay. This swiftly becomes internalized as shame—the belief that they are somehow defective. They learn that they can't trust majority people, that they will never be accepted for who they are."

Black's statement echoes what other survivors of color have personally shared with me. They say they feel too uncomfortable to talk about sexual abuse in a group where they question whether they can trust the majority of people to be understanding without regard to race.

These challenges, which seemed difficult in the early 1990s, seem even more daunting in 1997. A recent AP poll (1996) shows that 66 percent of African-Americans are pessimistic about the future because of the tense race relations that currently exist in the country. The media images surrounding both verdicts in the O.J. Simpson cases starkly demonstrate that in many instances, white Americans and African-Americans have very different views about the police and the criminal justice system; and also have great difficulty in understanding each other's *different* views. Other issues like the changes in welfare reform and affirmative action carry similar differences of opinion.

Another area of difference was covered in recent national news stories. They *identified the most segregated hour of the week* as that hour when many people attend their religious worship services. In this area, where it might appear that humans should be able to set aside differences and come together, there is the most separation. In one community, which has performed the Christian Passion Play for eighty-two years, the director received a death threat for casting a black man to play Jesus. They received numerous calls of complaint, some groups canceled their tickets, and others demanded that they be able to see the show with the "other Jesus," a white actor. All of this division in 1997 over a play about unconditional, universal love.

In this climate of difference, which sparks, at least, a feeling of discomfort and, at most, feelings of distrust; it is understandable that bringing groups of these people together to talk about the very personal issue of sexual abuse might be difficult at best. The sad reality, and my biggest fear, is that this social condition will work to prevent people of color—particularly African-American men—from seeking help through group work; merely because American society is not ready to face the truth about its past and how that affects the present.

The second external prejudice involves two sexual myths about African-Americans. One myth is that all men of color have enormous *sexual potency*. This myth often includes an assumption about penis size. The myth has its historical roots in slavery, when slaves were lined up like cattle before men, women, and children and publicly examined. Rumors began about the length of some male penises and the sexual potency of the *breeding* males. Though based on historical circumstances, various forms of this myth continue today. Some young African-American males unwittingly carry this myth as a badge of honor.

Women of color face the myth that they have great *sexual prowess* — almost animalistic. This myth, too, is rooted in slavery, where young women were forced to give birth as soon as they were old enough and then were bred like animals. The rumor spread that these women were very fertile and sexually proficient, and these women often were used as desired sexual objects by their masters. The proficiency myth has grown and transformed since those times, but it is still being fueled today through general social sexism and sexist advertising practices.

Many people today continue to take the *potency* and *proficiency* myths as fact and do not examine the history that created them. In fact, they are often joked about. In this climate, it is very difficult to face a group of people who might make statements like, "Well, black men are known to be hung, so why be surprised that they start having sex earlier." Or, "Black women are so sexy, who can blame someone for being attracted to them." I have actually heard such statements, often made about preteens and adolescents, more times than it is comfortable to admit.

As a male survivor of color, I had a terrible time overcoming the feelings that would well up in me when I wanted to speak of my abuse. After all, I was a male of color who was victimized by other males of color. How could I expect the other members of an all-white group to understand the feelings of guild, shame, and betrayal I felt at even mentioning that? How could I even indict my own race that way? What was my responsibility to my race?

Feeling the alienation of being a male of color in a society that had more stereotypes for me than I at first imagined, and being faced with sexual myths that were *supposed* to bring honor, I was initially trapped. External pressures threatened social emasculation and isolation if I revealed my abuse; and the internal pressure caused by keeping the silence made suicide seem like the only real way out. At times, the constant internal pain was worse than the thought of facing the unknown journey into death.

INTERNAL PREJUDICES

The most destructive internal prejudice I faced was simply internalizing the negative judgments of the larger society. Throughout my early childhood, I noticed that I was treated differently, and many times without respect. That fact, coupled with growing up in a culture that sometimes seemed to accept the negative stereotypes imposed upon it, was very confusing for me as a youngster. Coping with this inner confusion continues to be a lifelong struggle, especially with the escalating racial tensions evidenced in the media daily.

In my personal history, many factors fueled this internalized prejudice. Growing up in an alcoholic home where sexual abuse was present, I was taught the lessons of *don't talk*, *don't trust*, *don't feel*, *don't relax,* and *don't sleep*. Living below the poverty line in a segregated, southern housing project and constantly seeing that people of color were over represented among the unemployed, the underemployed, the undereducated, and the socially disabled left me feeling that we (people of color) were different and, somehow, severely damaged.

There were, and are, too few role models to sufficiently counter these early messages, which tend to be reinforced throughout one's life irrespective of high achievement. For example, when I was one of twelve persons of color in an entire law school, I recall hearing some classmates bemoan that they could not believe "they allowed niggers and Jews to come to this school."

I've discovered that many of us continue to replay our internalized, negative messages until we self-educate beyond them. For a survivor of color, this education is as much an integral part of recovery as dealing with sexual abuse issues. Recovery is about being honest with ourselves and about what actually has happened in our lives. A part of this process must include recognizing that racial prejudice is rooted in the historical development of American society.

Recognizing the role of race may help African-Americans understand how race issues become intertwined with our process of healing from sexual abuse, especially with our feelings of discomfort in groups. This acceptance is necessary for our personal growth, and it need not be argued or justified.

There is great social resistance, even today, against accurately examining how race has played a part in American history and in the social history of African-Americans. As survivors, we cannot wait for society to face these issues before we face them. They are already very present for us. We live them everyday.

In Studs Terkel's *Race*, Peggy Terry makes the following point:

> "To a certain extent we're all racists. Maybe not to the point of burning crosses, but we have attitudes that we don't recognize in ourselves. I know I'll never be free of it. I fight it all the time. It's things you've grown up with

all your life. I will never reach the point where I can sit with black people and be unaware of their being black. I'm always afraid I'm going to say something wrong, even with those I love and trust."

This type of honesty can serve as an excellent model for communicating about race in a group. Honest communication like this can help people of color and other group members bridge a gap that often is rooted more in history than in personal judgments. Knowing that some people are willing to be this honest makes it less difficult to take the step of entering a support group. Though there may be people in the group who cling to stereotypes, there may be a Peggy Terry, too, and that makes it worth taking the risk.

I can attest to the fact that once we get past the racial barriers, the similarity of the effects of sexual abuse on the human soul creates an enormous bond among those engaged in the process of recovery. For many survivors, there is no substitute for sharing among other human beings—without regard to race, gender, or class—who have also survived the horrors of sexual abuse. Getting there is difficult work, but our lives are worth it.

This is a complex process, and I don't want to oversimplify it. This topic deserves a book, but until then, maybe this article can give some guidance. As a person of color who has survived sexual abuse and has been in recovery for over ten years, I would advise all survivors—and those who care for them—to examine their own external and internal prejudices, and to honestly address them when they come up in their recovery. This is the only way to truly get in touch with our deeper selves and reclaim the lives we were born with the right to live.

◆ ◆ ◆ ◆ ◆

Those of us who are white must take up M. E. Hart's challenge to work on identifying and eradicating our own racism and standing up against racism whenever we encounter it. This must be done not only in support of survivors of color, but because it will help us —

because it is the right thing to do. For the same reasons, men must work on their sexism, heterosexuals on their homophobia, non-Jews on anti-Semitism, and so on. Doing so will not only make us better people, it will help make the world a safer, more welcoming place.

SAFE AND SUPPORTIVE PERSON(S)

In addition to support offered by counselors, therapists, organizations, and groups, there is widespread agreement about the importance of filling one's life with *safe, supportive individuals*, both *peers* and *professionals*.

> "...safe and trustworthy people who affirmed my positive qualities and gifts, listened with no intent to fix me, and allowed me *to speak what I needed to come to believe*." — Zandy, 44, New Jersey

> "...sharing with a few trusted others what was happening to me. To be able to say 'I really hurt bad' and not be judged — but just heard." — Ken, 44, Ontario, Canada

> "...having developed a relationship with another male that I could trust. This really was a resource to me because it gave me the opportunity to talk things through 'on the hoof' as things came up for me in therapy. The gift of this friendship enabled me to feel safe enough to allow the memories to return in full Technicolor rather than the grey memories I had developed to numb away the pain. Sharing the pain didn't make it hurt less, but what it did for me was really underline the value of contact with others — and I had largely limited this in my attempts to keep safe. From where I am now — excluding others is too much of a cost. Thanks, Pete — you really helped. — John, 33, Devon, England

While the emphases shift from one stage of recovery to another, the *need for support* remains significant. This is especially evident during the early and middle stages of recovery, where more than two out of three men write of people who made a difference.

> "...seeing other people confide in me as I disclosed the rapes I experienced." — Michael, 40, New Jersey

Outside of the therapeutic setting, far and away the single largest subcategory of safe and supportive individuals is the *survivor's spouse, significant other*, or *life partner*.

> "...support from my wife, and her 'nagging' for me to get help..." — Bob, 39, Pennsylvania

> "Joseph has been my constant and steady support for over thirty years. I could not have made it without him." — William, 62, South Carolina

> "...a very supportive wife...Despite her fears...she supported me in doing the work I needed to do, allocating tight funds to this work, and nudged me tenderly at times to pursue options I don't think I would have pursued without her support." — Olin, 42, Vermont

> "...support from my partner." — Jerry, 47, Nova Scotia, Canada

> "...my wife...was in my corner. When I first really started to recall the abuse (at the hands of my brother), we had just begun our lives together as husband and wife. I often ask myself if I would have survived as long as I have if she hadn't walked into my life." — Gregory, 37, Ontario, Canada

That so many individuals view their primary relationship as a major support in early recovery (three times as many as any other category) again demonstrates the necessity of *safe contact*.

> "...just to have someone to acknowledge my tears, and hold me." — Benn, 32, Georgia

Other relationships noted (in descending order of frequency) are *friend(s)*,

> "...my closest friends, to whom I disclosed regularly, as I recovered memories. Shame was the biggest issue and this was the best remedy." — Bob, 45, California

> "...a special friend. Someone with whom I knew I would be safe." — Steven, 26, New Hampshire

> "...a friend who listened and encouraged, and phoned me

day and night with love and support." — Michael, County Dublin, Ireland

family or specific *family member(s)*,

"...my closest relatives...they all stayed behind me in this process of healing/recovery..." — Svein, 60, Norway

"My mother initially provided the only sympathetic ears to my plight about my father. She was also the only other 'witness' to crucial events long past." — Ron, 32, Ontario, Canada

"My brother stood by my side." — Alejandro, 27, Argentina

"...parent's understanding and urging to seek therapy..." — Bob, 46, Ontario, Canada

nonspecified *supportive people*,

"...someone who knew what I had been going through and would go through. He believed and trusted me." — Brent, 35, Oklahoma

a *woman* or *women*,

"...a close female friend who provided me emotional support in the midst of my feeling suicidal and overwhelmed..." — Jim, 55, Michigan

"...many women who could relate to my pain and confusion." — Avoor, 48, Wisconsin

clergy or *spiritual director*,

"I spoke with a priest who became a very close and dear friend." — Geoff, 35, Pennsylvania

another *man* or other *men*,

"...and my three closest male friends with whom I first shared the fact that I was sexually abused as a child." — Jim, 55, Michigan

"...men like me, men who had felt the same pains, men who understand..." — Luis, 35, Colombia

teacher,

> **"...she saw that I was hurting and didn't walk away." —**
> **Jimmy, 23, Mississippi**

and *adopted* or *chosen family.*

> **"...my therapist, my partner, and my family of choice,**
> **because they believed me and gave me the space to**
> **grieve." — Sam, 26, Virginia**

> **"I created a family of friends who weren't going to let me**
> **down." — Matt, 20, Iowa**

It is especially important — in light of all the attention that has been paid to clergy abuse — to remind ourselves not to condemn every member of a group for the abuses of some. There are many members of the clergy who have been heroic in their protection of boys, healing work with victims and survivors, and struggles to make church hierarchy acknowledge and address the problem. Many survivors would not have made it without the help of such individuals. Just as there are abusers in every category, there are also allies. Understanding this helps make recovery possible. Being abused by a woman doesn't make all women unsafe. Having an abusive father doesn't mean that all fathers are abusive. It may not *feel* that way for a long time, but it is true. And learning this truth makes a huge difference. Like abuse, help and support can come from many (sometimes unexpected) sources.

Other relationship categories that receive a single mention at this early stage of recovery are *child, colleague, doctor, caring community, schoolmates, work supervisor, sponsor,* and an inspiring *celebrity.*

> **"...a colleague and friend who cofacilitated with me**
> **workshops on abuse for teachers and parents." — Ram,**
> **50, Manitoba, Canada**

> **"...a family doctor who took the time to seek a therapist."**
> **— Bob, 46, Ontario, Canada**

> **"Another source of strength was my Al-Anon sponsor who**
> **was the first person I told after my head exploded. He**
> **said that...he believed me and would do anything that he**
> **could to assist me on my journey." — William, 46,**
> **Arizona**

> **"I had written her; I poured out my emotions and feelings to her. Her written response to my letter was crucial to my recovery."** — Dennis, 50, Illinois

In addition to the categories listed above, a significant number of men note the importance of *other survivors* during the early part of their recovery.

> **"...only trusted victims could be relied on."** — CC, 45, Kansas

> **"...contact with other victims of abuse helped relieve the feelings of being alone."** — Brad, 43, Florida

> **"...if I use the name recovery from the time when I realized that incest was a proper name for my childhood, the contact with other victims/survivors was most important. For me it was like a religious experience, the feeling of belonging to a worldwide, invisible brother/sisterhood."** — Hamid, 52, Denmark

The role of *other survivors* is mentioned by over 10 percent of the men in early recovery; it increases as recovery progresses.

> **"I met this Catholic priest who was himself a survivor of sexual child abuse. We talked of our common experiences. It was a relief for me to meet someone who had experienced what I had experienced. I felt I was not alone anymore with my burden even though I had shared this before with other people."** — Daniel, 39, New Brunswick and Ontario, Canada

Most of the responses (more than half) don't specify the gender of the other survivors.

> **"...being with other survivors..."** — Fred, 38, Virginia

Of those who indicate gender, other *male survivors* are cited three times as frequently as female survivors. This may reflect how important it is for the child victim and adult survivor to learn that he is not the only male to whom this has happened.

> **"...other men whom I was able to respect for their integrity and honesty and willingness to be real..."** — Richard, 45, Massachusetts

> "Meeting a man who was abused by his mother [and having him] say to me what my mother did to me was sexual abuse. This validation started me on my healing path. Having a book by men, for men, describing the reality that both genders can be abusers and both genders can be victims. I feel so conditioned that only men can be sexual abusers; by reading other men's stories I feel more human; I feel less alone." — Bill, 38, Alaska

But the importance of connection with *female survivors* has made all the difference for some men.

> "...a woman friend who was also a survivor. She prepared the terrain by sharing her own experiences and validating that I also had my own past without forcing the issue." — Pierre, 28, New Brunswick/Nouveau-Brunswick, Canada

> "...a woman friend of mine who had gone through similar childhood experiences, and had, in recent years, recovered the memories. I had other people who were very supportive, but this particular woman KNEW firsthand exactly what the pain is and how awful it is. When it first hits you, the hours seem like days and the pain seems permanent. It stays for months and you feel it will never end. It's very scary. This woman told me that it would end. Things would improve and I could believe her. She had credibility for me and she gave me hope." — Murray, 41, Ontario, Canada

This book contains just two direct contributions by women, quite different from each other, and both important. Here is the first, a splendid example of survivors supporting one another without realizing they are doing so. **Mary, 40, Massachusetts,** is a brilliant writer, able to convey universal truths in her observations of everyday life. She shows how seemingly simple incidents can create profound effects. I'm particularly appreciative of this story of her meetings with Richard Hoffman through his writing and in person. She provides vivid portraits of the two of them, and the important ripples the encounters produced for both. No doubt many readers will be touched by this story. (Note: Mary is M1; M2 is Mary's therapist.)

"In the solitude to which every man is always returning, he has a sanity and revelations which in his passage into new worlds he will carry with him. Never mind the ridicule, never mind the defeat; up again, old heart! — it seems to say, — there is victory yet for all justice; and the true romance which the world exists to realize will be the transformation of genius into practical power." — "Experience." Ralph Waldo Emerson

Coach was showing the boy some 8-millimeter cartoons. The kind not meant for children—

Reading *Half the House* in one fell staring swoop, I realized that my out-of-service subway train has passed its last stop, headed for...Sunday night in the garage? 'Hello,' I called out. 'There's a person in here.'

Lights. Brakes. Startled driver. 'I'll swing around,' he said, and did.

Doors opened.

I got away. The boy in the book did not.

It started with M2's idea, sending me off to hear an author read from his new book.

M2: He's a kindred writer spirit for you. Cambridge library. Just go!

Your Recovery mentor says the next step is Cambridge, you go. At least it's closer than Lourdes. I packed mittens and applesauce and a drawing I made with a quote from Emerson. On the bus, I ate my snack and thought 'I'll go up and give him this drawing. Maybe then he'll say Hi, even shake my hand and talk about writing for a little.'

The librarians there were talking and laughing. One said, "Hello, looking for something?"

"Yes, sir, might I get some water before Mr. Hoffman reads? I don't want to be late."

"Certainly," he laughed. "I'm Richard. And we won't start without you."

He waited for me, then began to read. "It all depends on how deep your brothers are buried...."

My secret. He told the whole audience! Here for twenty-five years I've dreamed of crawling through old houses, digging for clues. (I'm probably the only client who came to M2 to talk about old-house architecture.) Finally the dreams became —

M1: They're a search for buried children. And it's up to me to remember where they are and how they died. But that's crazy! I don't want to waste your time talking about it.

M2: Cassandra! (He spoke very gently. As if talking to someone walking in their sleep.)

M1: Cassandra? Cassandra of Troy?

M2: Mm. Condemned to tell the truth, and to never be believed.

Truth? He *believed* me? I remember sliding to the floor, saying over and over, 'I think there's a problem. I think that something happened —' The real work began then.

Oh! But meanwhile, here at the library. Mr. Hoffman began to read about the Coach. Hm, was I ready to hear this? Nope. I tossed my drawing in front of him and ran for the bus.

M1: Aw, golly. So much for my chance to meet a kindred spirit! He must wonder why —

M2: Mary, no. He's a *Mensch*, Mary. He wouldn't wonder at all.

But M2 still had this bee in his bonnet, believing there are kindred spirits out there who would be happy to meet me. So he sent me to yet another Richard Hoffman reading.

Afterward I went up to Mr. Hoffman and said, "Hi, I bolted from a reading of yours —"

"Emerson," he says, and his eyes light up. "YOU left that drawing with the quote from Emerson. I showed it to everyone I know."

When you meet a famous person, you should probably not sink your fingernails into their shirt cuffs like I did then, no matter how amazed you are. "What? Really?"

"Then I sent a copy to my father as a step in mending our relationship. Because *Half the House* is really his story, too."

No matter how deep your children are buried, especially if one of them is you, don't dig by yourself. Go find allies. Just go. Pack applesauce and mittens. If you miss your stop, if cartoons loom in the dark, shout, "Stop this train. There's a person in here."

This time, somebody will listen.

Next time, the one who listens can be you.

A note to people who care about survivors: NEVER underestimate the importance of your caring. Even the smallest act of support, understanding, and love can have unimagined effects. *You do make a difference*. I have seen many examples of love's ripple effect. The preceding story by Mary is one of them. Here are three more:

> "...my son...made a profound statement to me, 'How the hell do you expect me to get better when you are ill?' He stated that I needed to be in treatment. I took his advice and went to...a seven-day inpatient program.... I didn't realize what I was in for. Two young men, during introductions, made a statement that they were there to deal with sexual abuse also. It hit home. I almost fell over.... I, for the first time in many years, got honest with myself and disclosed that I am an alcohol-dependent person and that I am a victim and survivor of sexual abuse. With the help of these two men I was able to deal with my sexual abuse and talk about it." — Gug, 46, Pennsylvania

> "...an initial suggestion from a friend who was/is a minister to 'go and talk to the school counselor.' From there I did check into the University's counseling, and it was *free* (and my parents never knew about it until I chose to confront them). I went to counseling for two and a half years at the University, both in group and individual therapy." — Chris, 22, Texas

> "Another person...was James, although his support would eventually become too much for him and we would drift

apart over the years that followed. Even now, I still think of him. If I ever were to say who was a true friend to me, his name would be the one I speak." — Gregory, 37, Ontario

WRITING ACTIVITIES

Writing is important to male survivors at every stage of recovery.

"...my own creativity. That creativity enabled me to devise an 'other world' where I could escape and live and grow up. It wasn't safe or pretty, but it sure as heck was better than what was happening to me in the real world. Years later (I am a writer), I was working on a short horror story about a group of young boys in an orphanage haunted by a rather demonic teddy bear. As I wrote, I realized that the real monster of the story was the Headmaster, who was sexually abusing the children. And through that story, my own real-life story (which I had somehow forgotten) came back to me. Today, I use creative writing to get in touch with my real feelings about the abuse and its effect on me at present." — Michael, 31, New York

A significant number of responses at all stages of recovery refer to some form of writing activity.

"...writing down in one place all the reasons, memories, and evidence that I had been incested. Early on, doubts would surface constantly, and I'd find myself thinking, *No, that's crazy; it couldn't have happened.* At such times. I couldn't remember the pieces that had convinced me that I was incested. Writing them down helped in a lot of ways. It showed me the shape of a pattern that snatches of memory didn't reveal. Also, I could sit down and read them, and believe all over again. Finally, just knowing that I had them all written down helped quench the doubts." — Olin, 42, Vermont

About half of these responses are fairly nonspecific, referring to *writing in general*, or keeping some form of *journal* or *log*.

"I found refuge in writing down thoughts, reminiscences, and reactions to things past. This process, for me, was an

> invaluable tool in acknowledging my past and validating my present." — Osvaldo, 41, Iowa

> "...a daily journal of my thoughts, memories, dreams, reactions — sort of homework between sessions." — Kristian, 52, Saskatchewan, Canada

> "I logged entries in my notebook every day. Seeing them there somehow let me know that my life was real." — Blaine, 40, Utah

Some men use writing because they are not yet ready to speak about the abuse.

> "Journal writing was a good resource early in recovery. I was able to write about feelings and memories even though I wasn't able to talk about them." — Tom, 36, New York

> "At first...I had to write the experiences as I was unable to speak the words due to the level of shame and pain." — Adrian, 45, Massachusetts

In addition to the general responses, early recovery entries in this category include composing a *personal history*.

> "...writing about and sketching traumatic events in my childhood. This process accomplished two things for me; it 'scaled down' the events in my mind, somehow diminishing the magnitude of them. It also, subsequently, gave me a sense of control — if the abuse was in a book, I could close it, burn it, throw it away!" — Kurt, 39, Georgia

Others speak of *writing to the perpetrator(s)* (whether or not these letters are actually sent), writing *songs* or *music*, keeping a *dream journal*, writing *fiction*, writing *to the Church*, and *letter writing*.

> "Write to other survivors." — Dennis, 50, Illinois

At a recovery weekend **Frank, 28, Virginia,** sang his own version of the traditional hymn "Amazing Grace," after adapting it to reflect the course of his recovery:

Amazing Grace

Amazing Grace, how sweet the sound
That saved a boy like me!
I once was lost, but now am found
Was numb but now I feel.

'Twas God that brought me here today
My spirit hurt, but alive!
How precious I am, and good to the core
I do believe today.

They all took from that little boy
But now I know their ways!
I will protect my little boy
No more shall he be hurt.

I still have work to do from here
But now it's work for me.
I've made it this far, I may even cry
For I am human too.

OTHER CREATIVE ACTIVITIES

Various forms of artistic pursuit may provide entry to recovery.

> "In *any form*, before I was able to speak about my incest
> experiences and sexual abuse, I found artistic expression
> to be my only true voice; sing, dance, write songs, paint,
> act, or whatever moves you. I write/perform my own
> songs. It saved my life." — Xandu the Giant, 33, New
> York

The process increases as recovery progresses. There are twice as many responses in this category by late recovery compared with the early and middle stages. I see this as evidence that once a survivor no longer needs to expend a significant amount of his attention and energy just to get through the day, his natural creativity and joy of living begin to blossom. Still, creative endeavors can be important during the early days of recovery. Responses in this category range from *general creativity* to various forms of *art,*

> *"...drawing pictures of my vague, distant feelings, when I didn't know what they were or couldn't name them. Also, noticing little beams of light — parts of melodies, songs, prayers, literature — which seemed to stir something in my dark numbness."* — Ira, 44, New York

> *"...painting and drawing, which allowed feelings and memories to surface."* — Mik, 40, Grand Cayman, British West Indies

music (including singing, playing instruments and listening to music — the specific music mentioned ranges widely, including Tchaikovsky's Sixth Symphony, Bach cello suites, Rachmaninoff, Dvorak, requiems, Cambodian *gamelan*, African drums, jazz, classical, and new age),

> *"...music. Lots of it, and lots of different kinds. I came to know myself and my full range of feelings by listening — all the time — to music...no lyrics, no other people's words, no words at all — just music.... Just physical and emotional experience undergone consciously this time. A kind of recalibrating the self's sensors, a spiritual retuning."* — Richard, 45, Massachusetts

> *"...music. It was the safest way for me to feel because it was solitary yet comforting."* — Tim, 32, Connecticut

> *"I could sing what I couldn't say."* — Will, 55, Arkansas

movement, *dance*, and *acting*.

> *"I began to move. First I only explored space. Later I danced."* — Wim, 28, Netherlands

Other activities listed include *roller skating, tai chi, baths, hugging, weight lifting,*

> *"...weight lifting [for] diminishing the rage and [increasing] empowerment."* — Iceman, 20, Illinois

noticing the environment, and *"staying put."*

> *"...living in the same city for more than three months..."* — Xandu the Giant, 33, New York

Taking Difficult but Necessary Steps

Person after person writes of taking actions necessary to his healing. As might be expected, the type of action changes over the course of recovery, but the courage displayed by these men remains constant. During the early stages of recovery, the most common responses in this category include first *acknowledging* or realizing that abuse has occurred,

> **"...believing that by acknowledging the childhood events as abuse, I would begin to heal. I relied on support from my therapist and my wife to reaffirm and believe this."** — Bob, 45, New York

> **"...to realize that there was abuse no matter how blanked out my mind is..."** — CC, 45, Kansas

and then *breaking the silence and secrecy.*

> **"I told someone I loved about what happened to me."** — George, 43, Nova Scotia, Canada

> **"For the first time I spoke out my pain loud and clear."** — Frank, 37, Idaho

> **"I told my good friend and he kept my secret until I was able to tell others."** — Max, 50, Netherlands

Since recognition of the abuse is a prerequisite for recovery, it isn't surprising that no one refers to it in later recovery. Silence and secrecy keep the abuse locked in place, so it makes sense that seven times more men mention breaking the silence during early recovery than in later stages.

> **"...confession, talking about who I am, what I struggle with."** — Robert, 46, California

> **"...being able to share my story of childhood in group psychotherapy."** — Jay, 40, Texas

As vital as recognition of the abuse and breaking the silence are to survivors, we must accept that they represent the *beginning* of a long process, not an end in themselves. And, like many aspects of recovery, they often have to be repeated. It can feel frustrating and discouraging to go back and repeat something that you thought you had completed. But if you examine the experience carefully, you will see that the meaning and impact are somewhat different each time; repetition can serve to reinforce, deepen and solidify your gains.

◆ ◆ ◆ ◆ ◆

These are the first lines of a poem of liberation by **Bobby, 31, Georgia**:

**Bobby's
"Declaration of Independence"**

**On a brisk fall day, many years ago,
My life was changed — on that day I said NO.
From nine to fourteen I was beaten and raped.
All I knew that day was I had to escape.
On that wonderful day I had found my voice.
I realized then that I did have a choice.
I regained control and was no longer ashamed.
I now understand that child wasn't to blame....**

◆ ◆ ◆ ◆ ◆

Many survivors emphasize that *remembering, recognizing that they were abused, telling someone* about it, *finding someone* who can listen, hear, and believe were steps that began the most important journey of their lives.

> **"...the desire to retrieve the memory of my childhood! Once I had resolved the issue of culpability and put the blame squarely where it belonged, a new perspective, unclouded by shame and guilt or distorted by fear, was mine. This realisation, that by excluding the painful from my memory, the positive experiences of childhood fell victim to the same censorship, was the key to unlocking a newfound respect and admiration for the courage of the child I was. As the poet Hardy said, 'If way to the Better there be, it exacts a full look at the worst.'" — Paul, 43, Devon, England**

> **"...first realizing that I had in fact been abused as my shame was clearly showing me...People were put in my path to whom I could begin to broach the subject of sex, sexuality, and abuse." — Bill, 49, Michigan**

"I admitted that it was not right." — Matsuo, 21, Japan

"...finding someone who is totally trustworthy and extremely understanding so I could begin to tell what happened to me as a child. This first courageous step is the most important on the dangerous road to recovery." — Michael, 43, Surrey, England

◆ ◆ ◆ ◆ ◆

This is an excerpt from the poem **"Repressed Memories"** by **John, 38, Alaska**:

With each day I feel the burden lifting.
> The burden of my secret.

Now I can tell my story.
Now I can let go of all the shame.
Now I can let go of the deep,
> deep,
>> deep,
>>> deep entrenched fear of being myself.

◆ ◆ ◆ ◆ ◆

After the crucial beginning — breaking the silence — there are many more miles to be traversed, one step at a time, in this journey of recovery. Other brave and difficult steps include *getting sober/abstinence* (from whatever addictive substances or behaviors are being used to numb feelings and distract attention from the pain),

"Not yet ready to face my sexual abuse issue, while dying from alcohol abuse, I first had to face my addiction(s) in a twelve-step recovery program. Once I achieved a length of sobriety (three years) and felt secure in this new way of living, I discovered the gift of courage to face my soul murdering childhood." — Brent, 48, Utah

"Getting sober...was the real beginning, but I did not start to intentionally address my abuse until I was sober five years." — Bill, 49, Michigan

"...admitting my drinking, recognizing my being in a self-pity mode, noticing my depression..." — Rodger, 31, Montana

> *"...becoming sober and then aware of how much of my self-abuse was related to childhood sexual abuse."* — Steven, 37, New York

telling or *sharing one's story, public speaking, coming out as gay,*

> *"...being open about my sexual orientation [which] allowed me to start talking about my childhood and the abuse I suffered."* — Rob, 33, Idaho

and having a *legal name change.*

> *"...and legally changed name. Gave me my own life back."* — Gary, 32, New York

When we look at the responses that address later recovery, we will see that, while specific steps may change, the bravery and strength of male survivors remain constant.

ATTENTION TO SELF

Throughout the healing journey, there are dramatic developments in the *relationship of the male survivor to himself.*

> *"...to put me first..."* — Stan, 47, Indiana

During early recovery, there is only a scattering of responses that emphasize the self.

> *"...to know that I was not alone and that I was not damaged goods — that I could be loved — to know that God cared and still loved me in spite of all that happened — to know that and discover that I had my own personal boundaries and to learn which side I belonged on."* — Mark, 34, Alberta, Canada

The numbers increase significantly by mid-recovery. Still later this category becomes a major focus. But at the beginning, the only aspect that receives more than a single response (two) is the survivor's own *inner strength.*

> *"When I believed in myself, my own strength surpassed that of every therapist I came across and even that of my best friends."* — Bob, 48, Illinois

> **"...my inner strength no matter how small..."** — Bob, 39, New York

Inner strength is not mentioned at all in later-stage responses when self-focus takes a different direction.

Other self-referential areas in the early days include taking *personal responsibility* and nonspecific self-focus.

> **"I accepted that I was responsible for what I made of my life and I stopped using the abuse as an [excuse] for why I was having problems now."** — George, 43, Nova Scotia, Canada

ATTENTION TO OTHERS

Here, too, there are extreme differences through early, middle, and late recovery. At the beginning of the process, a survivor's entire focus is on survival and personal recovery. Not one response to the first question refers to individuals, groups, or activities outside of these areas. As we see in the area of creativity, continuing progress frees healthy attention in directions beyond basic survival and recovery needs. Later, after more healing has taken place, the male survivor will be better able to give to others and take action in the wider world.

RELIGION AND SPIRITUALITY

In this area of life — as in others — there is significantly less focus (about half as much) during early recovery than later on. A few people refer to a *Higher Power, God* or "*The God Within*" in response to Question 1; a few more mention *prayer, devotions,* or *meditation*.

> **"...silently meditating, in groups and alone, gently noticing feelings and breathing, tears welled up softly as I knew I had been molested; others heard *and believed*."** — Lawrence, 62, New York

One man writes of *religious teachings* and another of *Native American spirituality.*

> *"...my friend...who helped to keep me connected with myself and others through Native American spirituality."*
> — Billy, 42, County Avon, England

Religion and spirituality are rarely mentioned by those who were abused by clergy or in a ritual context. There is usually a great deal of healing to be done before the survivor of ritual or clergy abuse can reclaim his spiritual life.

Donald, 50, Massachusetts, shares a very personal statement, one that he worked on, changed and polished for a considerable length of time until it was right for him. Here is a portion of his contribution:

This is my prayer and morning meditation.

God, I offer myself to thee — to build with me and to do with me as thou wilt....

When I put my pain in your hands and my will and my life in your care, you show me:

where I am loved, where I am manly, where I am enough, where I am nurtured, how you will keep me safe from dying for want of food or want of love, where I am esteemed and where I am valued. You replace my pain with serenity, you fill my emptiness with your warmth, you show me where I am worthy of being loved.

Help me to hold on to the vision that with your help I can abide the temporary discomfort of deprivation which is transitional out of pain and into peace.

...I cannot do this alone nor do I have to. When I do all the things I can, ask for your help and open myself to the flow of your spirit, you always do for me all the things I cannot do for myself.

Grant that I find the self-love today to treat myself with kindness and respect.

Show me the way, grant me knowledge of your will for me and the power to carry that out. Help me to remember that faith without works is dead. Direct my thinking away from self-pity, dishonest, or self-seeking motives. Grant me inspirations, decisions and intuitive thoughts. Help me to relax, take it easy and let you run the show.

Help me to live with myself, my pain, and my past.

Help me tolerate and live through my feelings.

Grant me willingness to change and the courage to heal today.

Grant me sobriety over sex and love addiction, abstinence from compulsive overeating, freedom from acting out...in what I do, what I say, and what I think.

Grant me recovery.

Thank you for your gifts.

◆ ◆ ◆ ◆ ◆

FEELINGS

Free expression of emotion is essential to healing, but can only occur after sufficient safety has been established. This may be why so few men speak of the role of feelings in early or even middle recovery. (We find impressive growth in this area later.) In answering the first question, only one person refers to *feelings in general*, and a few more to *crying* or *grieving*.

> **"The most important thing to me early in recovery was a safe place and safe person, and, I estimate, five hundred hours of hard crying (that comes out to six and a half full boxes of Kleenex)."** — Richard, 45, Massachusetts

The numbers actually diminish during mid-recovery — but then increase powerfully in the later stages. As survivors rediscover their full humanity, there is strong growth not only in the number of responses that deal with feelings, but in the *range* of emotions expressed.

◆ ◆ ◆ ◆ ◆

These are the first two stanzas of a poem by **William, 46, Arizona,** evoking the importance of expressing fears and feelings. In his accompanying letter, William wrote, **"I've enclosed a piece of my poetry that I believe speaks directly to the feelings that sur-**

vivors share.... I think that you have probably heard these sentiments from many others, and offer them as testament to my personal recovery."

Rainy Season

Sometimes it feels like
it rains inside my head.
It doesn't really bother
me, too much.
I'm almost glad
to have my thoughts cleansed.
They're easier to hold
that way.

Sometimes my body rains.
From my eyes, mostly.
But, at night,
it rains all over.
Like stuff just wants
to get out of me.
It feels like rain.

◆ ◆ ◆ ◆ ◆

INTIMATE RELATIONSHIPS AND OTHER AREAS NOT MENTIONED

The responses to Question 1 contain no mention of exploring intimacy, relationships, dating, sexuality, or nurturing. There is no talk of forgiveness, either of self or others. There is no mention of risk-taking, play, enjoyment, hope, or joy. There is no focus on the positive, the here and now, or plans for the future. The time of early recovery is hard. Survival — beginning to look at the issues and creating safety — doesn't allow for much else. The rest will come later.

For now, one individual mentions loving his *pet*.

"...this new puppy...is a living embodiment of love and trust and safety and when I need to cry she stands over me and keeps me safe. She is there day in and day out, loving me regardless." — Benn, 32, Georgia

◆ ◆ ◆ ◆ ◆

Keith, 31, Quebec, Canada, shares two metaphors of the recovery process — one in the form of prose, the other as poetry. Whether recovery is seen as wilderness survival (as in the following prose piece) or a small boat at the foot of a great waterfall (as in his poem "Maid of the Mist," which appears later), Keith's writing celebrates the rewards that make your efforts worthwhile:

When you are hiking, the heaviest, most essential, and most problematic component in your pack is drinking water. You can live for weeks without food, but a few days without water will leave you dead. Bacteria found in the lakes and streams of wilderness areas can leave you running through the woods, wishing you had listened when they said: "Don't drink the water." On long hikes, you should be carrying a minimum of a day's supply of water—two liters at least. And more in the summertime when perspiration takes its toll on dehydration. It is carried in half — and one-liter bottles, so that, if you break a bottle, you do not lose your whole supply. The bottles are refilled from streams and rivers that you pass along the trail. Whenever you come to a stream, you pull out the filter and fill all the empty bottles, even if the water is green and tastes foul. As it is filtered, it will not make you ill, and the taste can always be disguised with Tang or tea, but not drinking will make you sick for sure. You must carry it because you never know where the next stream is, or what condition it is likely to be in. Even if the topographical map shows a river, it may be dry, or have relocated, or taste worse than this one does. When you do arrive at a stream that is running cool and clear and sweet, you take out all your bottles and drink again. Then you load up your pack and carry on to the next stream, the next camp, the next mountain.

And now we move on to "the next stream, the next camp, the next mountain."

Part Two

MID-RECOVERY

The second question addresses a further point in the recovery process. It reads:

"As my recovery progressed, I found help and encouragement from..."

Once again, I indicated no specific time frame, to allow for as much freedom as possible in the responses.

BOOKS AND READING

In mid-recovery, compared with the early stages of healing, only two-thirds as many men cite books and reading as sources of *help* and *encouragement*. However, books and reading remain crucial to many survivors for *information* and *connection*. This is especially true for men who are more isolated geographically or socially.

> **"A friend told me of your book. It took three months to get it. It was for me a lifeline." — Jose, 41, Argentina**

> **"...all of the statements by fellow survivors that were exactly the way I also felt." — Mike, 37, Prince Edward Island, Canada**

> **"...connecting with the experience of others thro' books mainly..." — Mik, 40, Grand Cayman, British West Indies**

Some are not yet ready to move beyond this protective environment.

> **"I found help and encouragement from books, which were easier to approach than people because I was embarrassed and, I guess, ashamed about what happened." — Michael, 31, New York**

For others, however, the role of books has changed. As recovery progresses, isolation decreases. New resources take on greater importance. Perhaps as a result of what he learned from his reading, the survivor begins to explore the external world.

> **"I read of a world I did not know. I explored first in my imagination.... Then, travelling." — Kemal, 48, Turkey**

Survivors are increasing their ability to risk moving out of a small protective circle into a larger environment, and books and reading are mentioned less frequently. But many men continue to note their significance as companions and guides on their journeys.

> **"...reading about the experiences of others." — Phillip, 48, Kentucky**

> **"Through reading books directly about incest and books related to issues of survivors, I began to confront, feel, and move beyond the remaining tendrils of the abuse." — Jim, 26, Massachusetts**

Some of the books that were mentioned in early recovery are now listed by the same people as continuing sources of support. Some of these same books are being newly discovered by survivors as they explore a literary world beyond their own experience. Still other works are new additions to the list.

Unlike the answers to Question 1, the greatest number of mid-recovery responses are nonspecific, referring to *reading*, *books*, or *learning*. The number of individuals who fall into this subcategory is slightly higher now.

> **"...reading many books. Opening my mind and heart to new understanding." — Julian, 30, Hong Kong**

> **"...all the books I read...I bought and read everything I could find. Hundreds of books!" — Brent, 35, Oklahoma**

> **"...books, journals, magazines...all the time reading." — Thomas, 45, Germany**

> **"I had much to learn. The information had long been kept hidden from me. I would let nothing keep me from the truth." — Stefan, 51, South Africa**

Once again, *Victims No Longer* is cited far more than any other book, but only about half as frequently as during early recovery.

> "*Victims No Longer* continued what *The Courage to Heal* had begun, an understanding that my life was getting better." — Ramesh, 40, India

> "...has given me the encouragement I needed and the education to push forward..." — Gug, 46, Pennsylvania

> "...gave to me the structure and direction necessary for my work." — Ryszard, 22, Poland

> "Sometimes I returned to the book to find that the information had new meaning to me." — Carlos, 47, Peru

The only other books that are cited more than once (twice each) are both new to the list. They are *The Courage to Heal Workbook* by Laura Davis and *Trauma and Recovery* by Judith Herman.

> "...the Laura Davis workbook...was like having a teacher and a friend when I was alone." — Alejandro, 27, Argentina

Three books listed in response to Question 1 are cited once in answer to Question 2. They are *The Courage to Heal, Repressed Memories*, and *Abused Boys*. In addition to these old friends, there are single mentions of fifteen★ books or authors. They are:

Bastard Out of Carolina by Dorothy Allison

Secret Survivors by E. Sue Blume

John Bradshaw (no specific work mentioned)

Healing Your Aloneness by Erika J. Chopich

How to Survive the Loss of a Love by Melba Colgrove

Soul Survivors by J. Patrick Gannon

Fire in the Belly by Sam Keen

Wendy Maltz (no specific work mentioned)

A Male Grief by David Mura

★ Sharp-eyed readers may notice that there are sixteen items on this list of fifteen. That is because one person cited *The Inner Child* without reference to an author. When I went to the library to check references, I found two books with the words "Inner Child" in the title, the works by Chopich and Taylor. So I included them both. If you are interested, you are welcome to check out both of them to see whether either speaks to your needs.

Out of Hell by Joe S.
The Little Prince by Antoine de Saint-Exupéry
The Inner Child Workbook by Cathryn L. Taylor
The Color of Light by Perry Tilleraas
Embracing the Journey by Nancy W.
Paddle Whispers by Douglas Wood
The Healing Woman (periodical)

In addition to reading books, several men say that *Internet/World Wide Web/On-Line* resources were of significant value during the middle part of their recovery.

> "...reading resources such as [*Victims No Longer* and *Abused Boys*] and being able to recognize parts of myself in the reported experiences of others. I also made individual contact with a few men through the Internet (the alt.sexual.abuse.recovery newsgroup). Typically these were very intense, detailed, and personal exchanges which allowed us to give appropriate support, affirmation, and perspective to one another over a period of particular need. I still correspond with a couple of these 'electronic friends' although I only read a.s.a.r. very sporadically and selectively now." — Kristian, 52, Saskatchewan, Canada

> "I continued to grow and share in IWA (I Was Abused section of Human Sexuality Forum on CompuServe) and after being there for about a year, the Section Leader resigned and I was offered the position. Being the Section Leader helped in my recovery a great deal." — Doug, 33, California

> "In support of my sexual abuse issues: the people on alt.sexual.abuse.recovery who accepted me, my story and my pain as real. They also helped to show me that I was not alone in my struggles.
>
> "In support of my struggles with D.I.D. [Dissociative Identity Disorder]: All the wonderful people on alt.support.dissociation who helped me to understand that I was not alone." — Warren, 31, Ontario, Canada

As access to computers increases, more and more survivors are making connections and locating information through the Internet. This is particularly true of younger individuals and those who are relatively isolated from direct access to other survivors or resources. Initially, the computer can provide an important way of reaching out of isolation for people who are not yet ready to risk more direct contact. Please remember that, like the real world, "virtual reality" has its share of frauds, manipulators, and dangerous individuals. By maintaining safe boundaries and taking reasonable precautions, you may find significant resources through your computer.

SAFE ENVIRONMENTS

Although the numbers decline quite a bit (by about half) from early recovery, several mid-recovery responses stress the importance of a *safe physical environment*. They are split between nonspecific references to a *safe place* and *residential treatment centers*.

> **"...a place of safety. A place to breathe." — Sam, 31, Nigeria**

> **"...a treatment centre for eating disorders and sexual abuse. My experiences there propelled me forward in healing, learning, and health building. I was able to do much work on myself and my issues. It gave me the physical and mental stability to be able to deal with my primary issues more specifically." — John, 32, Newfoundland, Canada**

In mid-recovery references to hospitals and drug/alcohol rehabilitation centers disappear. Perhaps by this point, survivors have achieved sobriety, understanding of their situation and some stability in their lives; they now require safe settings to work on their abuse recovery.

PROFESSIONAL RESOURCES

Professional *counseling* or *therapy* continues to be viewed as crucial in this middle recovery stage, although the emphasis shifts significantly.

> **"...increased therapy sessions..." — Stephen, 34, California**

> **"...my sobriety led to my therapy." — Magnus, 37, Sweden**

> **"...psychotherapy that focused on the childhood trauma: 1) made it real, 2) gave me permission to feel it and talk about it." — Doug, 57, California**

> **"In the early part of my recovery I was afraid of my therapists. I am now learning to trust them; I know they can help me." — Rodger, 31, Montana**

While the number of references to *individual counseling* and *therapy* remains constant throughout the recovery process, during mid-recovery there is a slight decline in the number of men who refer to their *individual therapist* or *counselor.*

> **"...working with my individual therapist, who was able to help me understand the meaning of my sexual 'acting out' and put that behavior in its proper perspective." — Sean, 29, Massachusetts**

This decrease might indicate that the survivor is shifting responsibility for his life from another person back to himself — a trend that continues in later recovery. Although counseling and therapy remain important resources, their centrality to the survivor's life is diminishing. The role of therapy (and thus the therapist) is evolving from a lifeline to a tool that can be employed when needed. A number of the responses now concern specific qualities of the therapist or aspects of therapy that have been particularly *helpful* or *challenging.*

> **"...therapists with good experience and understanding." — Rick, 35, Montana**

> **"...a warm, caring, sensitive person who is willing to listen and try to help me..." — Scott, 43, Brazil**

> **"...was a good listener and served as a sounding board." — Avoor, 48, Wisconsin**

> **"...psychodrama. It was extremely painful, but also extremely helpful to turn my anger away from myself and toward my abuser(s)." — George, 61, Washington State**

> **"...working with a therapist who is the same gender as my abuser (female). While this was initially too frightening, it became the most direct route to accessing my pain and longing." — Tim, 32, Connecticut**

> "...he resembled my father, but his heart was kind." — Ismail, 40, Malaysia

> "I sought out a private male therapist who was trained in addiction psychotherapy and once I trusted this man, I began to tell someone outside of me of the horrible and terroristic murdering of my inner child's soul. The therapist sent me to the Intermountain Sexual Abuse Clinic, which to that point has historically treated *only* women, for focused deep-level therapy. This was the most painful time of my recovery since my abuser was my mother, a woman possessed, and my recovery depended upon the guidance and support of a woman therapist and twelve other women in recovery." — Brent, 48, Utah

An important aspect here is the establishment and maintenance of *appropriate boundaries*.

> "...an individual woman therapist who one day said to me, 'No matter what happens in here we will never have sex.' I felt a geological shift deep down. Safety first." — Paul, 36, Pennsylvania

There is impressive growth in the category of *group therapy*.

> "...therapy, both individual and group. I learned I wasn't alone in my fears, anger. I wasn't unique; it was OK to be afraid, to be angry, and share those feelings with others who understood me...to howl, to cry, and find that I hadn't flunked life." — John, 58, Washington, D.C.

> "...to a therapy group conducted by my therapist, where I might risk a little more." — Peter, 43, South Africa

Unlike early recovery (Question 1 elicited four times more references to individual than to group therapy), mid-recovery responses focus more on group work than individual counseling. It is heartening to see male survivors opening themselves to wider circles of understanding and support.

> "...group therapy cannot be underestimated." — Bob, 43, Maryland

> "The range of responses available to me as a result of (the group) allowed me to tell my story and begin to notice

> that — despite (my) feeling dirty — others still found that they wanted to feel close to me for who I was. This encouragement has enabled me to challenge some of the beliefs that I held about myself and others." — John, 33, County Devon, England

Male survivors have started to gain trust in their peers.

> "...to be together with men. To help, not to hurt." — Luis, 22, Costa Rica

> "...being in men-only groups hearing each others' stories without uninvited comment or touching, helped heal my fear of sexual molesting by men...later, mixed-gender groups gave me heartwarming acceptance by women-survivors as a comrade." — Lawrence, 62, New York

Men, encouraged by competent counselors, are diminishing overde-pendence on a single individual. Their therapist is no longer seen as a "savior" or magician, but as a helper, teacher, guide — or caring friend.

> "...my therapist (new). It still seems [incredible] to me that talking with a man about my innermost thoughts and feelings (...I can now say that I actually have them!) could elicit such profound change." — John, 49, Massachusetts

> "...stands with me." — Teishiro, 34, Japan

At this point, for many male survivors, individual therapy is a home base from which they move to explore the wider world. The group setting has become an important laboratory — a safe (although sometimes scary) setting for practicing skills of relating to others.

> "Before I joined the group I was always a loner. I never knew how to talk to people and the only way I could relax was home alone. Now I can finally see why being around other people is a good idea. Group therapy with a good leader and the support of my group really helped me get there." — Terry, 49, Tennessee

> "...the safety and warmth of the group process." — Alford, 55, Minnesota

By mid-recovery, there is a significant increase in all of the subcategories of *group therapy*:

General/nonspecified (more than three times as many references as before),

> "...group therapy. I never knew that there were others like me." — Todd, 32, New York

> "...a mixed sex group. Though I was the only male at times, the interaction and open truth of everyone was really enlightening as I was not alone in my pain." — George, 61, Washington State

survivors' groups (four times as many),

> "...a group or groups that can be 'family'; other survivors are best." — Pete, 49, New York

male survivors' groups (over twice as many),

> "I joined a men's group for survivors of sexual abuse. It was an environment in which I could learn for the first time, as an adult, to trust another man. Men who have been sexually abused in their childhood by men still need men in their lives. The group setting was a good place to begin to allow men back into my life. I also have a need to venture beyond the group setting and learn to develop relationships with men in the larger community. — Geoffrey, 32, Colorado

> "...a male recovery group which met once a week. I think the experience of meeting with a group of men once a week to talk about our painful childhood issues has prepared me to expect encouragement and validation from men. I anticipate genuine responses from men, and am able to give them in return. I enjoy my son and daughter's company so much now. I believe these are the result of feeling like I belong in the company of men." — Ed, 46, Minnesota

> "...I joined a series of men's counselling groups on sexual abuse. My experiences there were so positive that today I recommend to all newcomers to find a men's group

and join. I believe that you cannot recover from sexual abuse without developing trust in your fellow man and finding love and acceptance in them. A survivors' group for men, facilitated by counsellors, is a wonderful, cheap, intense, and effective way of doing it." — John, 32, Newfoundland, Canada

"I worked through much of my anger in a nurturing, safe place." — Roger, 44, Florida

"...the ongoing Male Survivor Group continues that environment of safety and accountability." — George, 61, Washington State

"It felt wonderful to spend time with these people. They are my brothers." — Murray, 41, Ontario, Canada

and *men's groups* (twelve times!).

"...a group of other men, some survivors, some not..." — Dale, 42, Hawaii

"Men! The scariest animal of all. My men's group made it a lot less scary." — Van, 41, Colorado

The significance of this increase cannot be ignored. It provides continuing evidence that recovery occurs in the company of others. Humans are not meant to be solitary or isolated. As the survivor's wounds begin to heal, he reclaims his human nature as a social being — part of a larger community. For many men, group work is a key step in this process.

"...my group members...gave me support and stability in my recovery..." — Fred, 20, New Jersey

"Never could I have done this solo." — Juan, 67, Spain

"...the search for a survivors' group therapy that matched my needs and expectations." — Oliver, 53, Massachusetts.

Now, in mid-recovery, when we include references to all forms of professional therapy — individual and group — we find them in well over half the responses. This trend is reinforced by more than twice as many responses referring to *workshops* and *retreats*.

"...attending workshops where I learned my shame and pain was not unique. It was comforting to know that I was not the first person to relive my traumas in violent sexual fantasies, and realize that acting out was a defense used by many victims." — Adrian, 45, Massachusetts

"...a *wonderful* workshop...which was very beneficial in helping me place the responsibility of the abuse where it belonged, allowing me to focus more on my recovery." — Gene, 59, Washington State

"It was important to see that other men were suffering like I was. At that workshop I met (another male survivor who) informed me that there was a men's support group.... Back home, his group accepted me.... The communication is very healing to one who has been alone with his fears for so long." — Dan, 34, Ontario, Canada

"...a weekend retreat...planted the seed of my recovery and gave me roots, a network of support." — Bill, 38, Alaska

"...my experience in retreat weekends kept me going..." — Dale, 42, Hawaii

"...provided me with a space to out my abuse within a context similar to the one in which it had originally occurred, but of course the contradiction was that now it was completely safe..." — Barry, 24, New York

"The weekend was wildly wonderful and fruitful for me.... I loved every single guy there." — Donal, 41, New York

"I typically stifle exuberance, but the word that keeps running through my mind is 'amazing'...an amazing weekend. I found it affirming and life-giving." — Frank, 34, New York

◆ ◆ ◆ ◆ ◆

This poem is offered by **Pete, 36, New York,** in recognition of the support of other men at a workshop. They stood by him during a time of painful feelings and memories:

With these men I walked through the Cold Winter Storm,
And ate the flesh of my own soul.

> With these men I came to sing my song,
> And tell them what I know.
>
> My feathers were wet; my feet were bloody,
> But these days have all gone by.
>
> I ask of them now, these frozen men,
> To thaw, so we may die.
>
> Die to the past, these pains and sorrows,
> The horrors of all this loss.
>
> So that we may true, become anew,
> And live — to live — Alive.

As the survivor continues to recognize, acknowledge, accept, and appreciate the allies in his life, his world grows larger and larger.

> **"I found help and encouragement from the awareness of connecting with men and women survivors as people. They no longer were identified by their sex (male or female) or sexual orientation (homosexual, lesbian, straight), or as 'Christian' or 'non-Christian.' These 'people' became real people: persons recovering from sexual abuse with varying journeys. On my first weekend (workshop), my deepest experience was with a gay man named Dave who could share and identify with my pain at that point in my life. We embraced tenderly at the end of the weekend as men. He felt it ironic that his closest connection was with a straight guy. I thought it ironic that (mine) was with a gay man. The point was that we were beyond 'gay' or 'straight'...and we were just men. This encounter changed my life." — Zandy, 44, New Jersey**

The first two questions elicit equal numbers of references to *peer organizations*, *meetings*, *programs*, and *principles*, but once again the particular emphasis shifts from early recovery. This may be in response to a new focus in the survivor's life.

> **"...going to meetings. Working my program. Even when I didn't believe in it. Just showing up..." — Tom, 61, Maine**

> **"...integrating therapy with the twelve-step principles of spirituality." — Jay, 40, Texas**

During mid-recovery, the most frequent references are to *SIA/ISA* (Survivors' twelve-step) groups (a slight increase over early recovery),

> **"...about six months into my recovery I joined SIA. It was a hard step initially, because I would be meeting real people face-to-face. Being involved in SIA has been a key element in my recovery." — Doug, 33, California**

> **"...attending Incest Survivors Anonymous meetings. Here I found the loving and caring support from other victims. I realized I was not the only person that was degraded so terribly. In these meetings I met people that understood my feelings, emotions, and concerns. They all were so supportive." — Dennis, 50, Illinois**

followed by unspecified *twelve-step programs*, then *AA* (a slight drop), *V.O.I.C.E.S. in Action* (an increase), and *Al-Anon* (also an increase).

> **"Meetings of Alcoholics Anonymous led to individuals who had been similarly abused. This open discussion with trustworthy persons helped me a great deal." — John, 61, Maryland**

> **"The only encouragement I had was other victims' success. I have used 'VOICES' groups." — CC, 45, Kansas**

> **"...my Al-Anon men's group, to whom I disclosed, offered acceptance, compassion, and a forum for my thoughts. I went there when I did not feel safe." — William, 46, Arizona**

Next in frequency are *The Linkup* and *S.N.A.P.* (for survivors of clergy abuse), *ACA* and *ACOA*, and *NA* (Narcotics Anonymous).

> **"...where I learned to trust other people, and who shared their experience." — Stan, 47, Indiana**

There are several mentions of *men's groups*.

> **"...a men's group where I personally met and talked to other survivors." — Greg, 39, Indiana**

> **"...my weekly men's group continues. Some of the first participants have come back from time to time to check in, and then go back out into their lives again — refreshed that they are OK." — Bill, 45, Delaware**

> *"...close male friends' support group (not all survivors)..."*
> — Fred, 38, Virginia

> *"...although the group was only a short-term thing, I still find parts of healing from it."* — Jeff, 43, Nova Scotia, Canada

Other groups, each cited by one person, include *SLAA, CodA, Focus, SASAM, Catholic Family Services, Lutheran Family Services,* and *Families Anonymous.*

> *"...friends that I met at SASAM who also had been sexually abused. It helped me to know that I wasn't the only person that this had happened to."* — Dwayne, 44, Texas

> *"One counselor especially [at Catholic Family Services]...may not have realised it, but she was the first who helped me to understand that a child could not possibly be blamed for what had happened to him. And it was not wrong to be angry with my brother."* — Gregory, 37, Ontario, Canada

> *"...an informational group at Lutheran Family Services...was very helpful in aiding me to forgive myself..."* — Gene, 59, Washington State

> *"...these people [Families Anonymous] gave me the support I needed to deal with other family problems and gave me strength to 'look at myself.'"* — Dennis, 50, Illinois

Within the *twelve-step* category, one individual refers to a *group specifically for gay male survivors* and another writes about a *combined focus.*

> *"...Triple Winners twelve-step group...combines incest recovery with food and sex issues. It was the first time I could be completely honest in a twelve-step group setting."* — Michael, 30, Ohio

Participation in groups with other survivors is enormously important, meeting a whole range of needs.

> *"...being part of a group discussing sexual abuse issues and what kind of family I lived in."* — Charles, 45, Illinois

> "...attending support groups and listening to other survivors take a risk and share their secrets. Their courage gave me the boost in courage that I needed to take similar risks. I did!" — Bob, 45, New York

> "The first group I attended was for male and female survivors. Through attending, I found a group for males that met on a different night. I attended both meetings because they offered me different benefits. The mixed meeting let me see how pervasive abuse was on all economic levels. Whether the families were rich or poor, large or small, abuse had happened to the children living in them. I then started to see sexual abuse as a family, community, and ultimately a national problem. The all-male meeting helped me work on issues of truth and emotional honesty on a different level. I had multiple abusers, male and female. The majority were males. Because of the abuse, I had developed a lifelong trust problem with other males. The meeting helped me work on honesty and developing male camaraderie within an emotionally safe framework. So I could work on breaking down that trust barrier at my own pace, with other males who understood what I was going through." — Paul, 34, Washington, D.C.

When we add together all the therapeutic, group and organizational categories, it is easy to see that by mid-recovery an expansion process has taken hold.

> "...an agency for women who organized a conference for survivors and realized the importance of including men, as sexual abuse is a community problem and not a gender issue. They stood by their word that sexual abuse is not about sex but about power." — Pierre, 28, Nouveau-Brunswick/New Brunswick, Canada

The survivor never again has to retreat into isolation.

SAFE AND SUPPORTIVE PERSON(S)

Here again, as recovery progresses, we have ample evidence of male survivors opening their lives to *other people*.

"...other men and women, straight and gay, whose stories made my story come alive...they unlocked my closet door and helped me out into the light." — Peter, 37, Massachusetts

"...other friends whom I seemed to be meeting not only in AA, but also in Adult Children of Alcoholics and Al-Anon. I told one person, then another, and then at a group meeting, and then at an open Al-Anon meeting. Each time I felt freer, more empowered, and safer to speak out about what I had been holding onto. My recovering friends became my support group, letting me become more and more free." — Bill, 49, Michigan

"...other survivors and friends and family, who listened to my story and told me their own. Just speaking the unspeakable helps to release incredible amounts of energy. It helps make manageable old memories of trauma that at first seemed too horrible to encounter." — Olin, 42, Vermont

"...learning I was not alone, that there was help, that there was recovery. But, most of all, the really scary fact that some people care." — Ken, 44, Ontario, Canada

Overall numbers within this category have risen, and again the emphasis has shifted. While a significant number of men still list *spouse*, *lover*, or *life partner*, the numbers have dropped so that it no longer is the largest subcategory.

"...good therapy. Friends, who mostly proved to be extremely loving and patient. The most important resource during this period was my lover, although I didn't believe that at the time. He helped me understand how deeply incest had hurt me, and watched me fall apart. Fortunately, he was also there to support and challenge me — I think his unconditional love was the answer." — Jim, 35, Maine

"...my wife, who was and is patient with me — I'll never know why." —Timothy, 37, Alabama

"...a very supportive spouse. I do not believe my recovery would have been possible without her loving and caring support." — Dennis, 50, Illinois

> "...my lover...nothing would have happened without [him]." — Doug, 46, New York

This category of "significant other" drops to third place, in favor of a huge jump in references to *friend(s)* (four times as many as in the earlier stage),

> "...a little later, as I became more confident and less embarrassed, from close friends..." — Osvaldo, 41, Iowa

> "...friends. Sometimes you just need a hug." — Benn, 32, Georgia

> "...a few carefully chosen friends." — Barrett, 40, New Jersey

> "...a very good friend...provided the first male I could trust talking about the painful memories. He's been going through the same shit vis-à-vis his dad." — Ron, 32, Ontario, Canada

> "...a supportive and understanding special friend [who] flowed with my mood swings and helped to keep me mentally present and in touch with my emotions and above all, believed in me." — Curt, 43, Wisconsin

and *family* or *family member(s)* (almost a threefold increase).

> "...my wife and family, the people I most wanted to hide my ugly secret from." — Gene, 32, California

> "...my sister who suffered alongside me all those years." — Scott, 41, Michigan

> "...another family member who had gone through sexual abuse. When I started to give up, I thought about how they were fighting it in order to gain some measure of control over their life and [I] drew strength from that." — David, 35, Wyoming

> "My mom was as supportive as much as she was able to then." — Gregory, 37, Ontario, Canada

> "...one of my relatives who believed me..." — Douglas, 45, Czech Republic

The circle of trust is widening.

> "...friends outside of my program and some family members who were also in recovery, and meeting more and more survivors who would share their stories with me."
> — Dan, 28, Massachusetts

> "...one man I could trust, then another, and still another..."
> — Mohammed, 42, Pakistan

This expansion is further demonstrated by the appearance of a new category — *body worker(s)*. For a survivor to allow himself to be touched is evidence of a huge leap of trust. Willingness to engage in some sort of *body work* (responses include massage, *shiatsu*/acupressure, and chiropractic) represents significant risk-taking.

> "I also found touch therapy very useful to get in touch with my buried feelings." — Tom, 36, New York

> "...gentle massage therapy. I learned that touch can be safe. It doesn't have to be sexual." — David, 27, Oregon

Next come the subcategories of *nonspecified safe persons* (a slight decrease) and a slight increase in *caring community* or *support network*.

> "...others who would not harm me." — J.V., 28, Kenya

> "I found myself surrounded with love." — Max, 50, Netherlands

Only half as many now mention *clergy*,

> "...a V.A. [Veterans' Administration] chaplain...opened his arms to hear my pain, to 'listen' to my story. He gave me a spiritual foundation for recovery and growth from the devastation of self-destructive behaviors." — Mark, 34, West Virginia

and there is only one mention in each of the subcategories of *adopted* or *chosen family, doctor, other men, colleague,* and *children*.

> "...my wife of eleven years, but most importantly, my three primary aged children, through them I was able to see how vulnerable I was. I am also able to catch up with my lost childhood through playing and learning with them." — Christopher, 33, Victoria, Australia

> "I also owe a lot to my special friend at work whom I trusted to talk about my abuse, and his honesty in saying, 'I don't know anything about sexual abuse, but I'm your friend and I will listen.' He told me I'm OK — it wasn't my fault." — Gug, 46, Pennsylvania

In keeping with the trend toward increased social interaction, we see greater awareness of the importance of *other survivors*.

> "...other survivors. It's great to hear, 'I know what you're feeling.'" — Angelo, 25, Massachusetts

> "...they had known the pain. They knew of what I knew." — Klaus, 56, Switzerland

> "...no one else speaks to me and understands me the way another survivor does. There is always an instant connection, which at first was very scary." — Larry, 32, New York

> "... *Victims No Longer*, A.A., fellow survivors, wife, therapy, but mostly hanging out with my fellow survivors and *knowing I was not alone*!!!" — John, 38, Oklahoma

While the number citing *female survivors* remains small, and there is only a slight increase in references to *male survivors*, those who list *other survivors* without specifying gender grow by a third.

> "...a female friend (who) had also been abused and understood." — David, 61, Michigan

> "...other trusted male survivors, either one on one or in a group..." — Doug, 35, California

> "...other recovering people." — Colin, 33, California

> "...anyone who had had an experience anywhere parallel to mine. The personal histories in *Victims No Longer* were an important element." — Bob, 65, Delaware

> "...just being around other survivors that told me that I certainly was not the only male survivor around, and especially that there is life after incest — that there is a wonderful, productive life that does not have a black veil of shame and secrecy over every part of it. There is really a joy to being *me* and a reason to keep on living." — Chris, 57, Ohio

When I compared the answers to Questions 1 and 2, I found roughly the same number of men writing about other people, both professionals and nonprofessionals. However, by mid-recovery, decreased emphasis on professional support is balanced by greater importance of *nonprofessionals* in the survivor's life.

> "...people who were big enough to *witness* and validate my experience." — Dale, 42, Hawaii

A fairly substantial new subcategory raises the numbers even further — references to *hearing other survivors' stories*.

> "...listening to the stories of other survivors, I started to take my own story seriously." — Rod, 48, Rhode Island

> "...other survivors telling their story. Their story was my story." — Jimmy, 23, Mississippi

WRITING ACTIVITIES

The importance of writing remains constant throughout the recovery process, with some shift of emphasis. The largest category remains *nonspecific*, *journaling*, or keeping a *log*.

> "...my journal kept me centered and focused." — Patrick, 42, Rhode Island

> "I found writing most helpful in both exploring hidden memories and gaining insights.... I MUST know what happened. Trying to cover over the experience is the root of denial.... I have always felt a compulsion to write; now I know why." — John, 43, County Mid Glamorgan, Wales

The next largest subcategory, a new entry, is writing *poetry* — offering further indication that the survivor's frozen creativity is thawing.

> "My poetry and prose is not all about abuse, yet somehow it is, as the issue is expressed in many different ways in my writing. I have some that I share, and some that I don't even read myself. I have saved most; some have been sent in letters to special friends." — Keith, 31, Quebec, Canada

> "I looked inside myself and there I found the poet I never knew I was." — Jürgen, 36, Germany

"I am proud of them, like they are my children...they come from inside me. And some people have been touched by one or the other of them. That is affirming for me. For me to express myself is what they are all about. The very idea of having to do 'creative writing' used to strike me with terror or at the very least seem impossible. And somehow in all my years of education I managed to avoid it. I think that stifled my technical and analytical writing, putting it in a straitjacket. After all, things like feelings could not come out.... After all, I think I have been getting my voice back." — Larry, 44, Pennsylvania

Here is an excerpt from one of Larry's poems:

Childhood

Laughter and giggles,
Warmth, caring and love,
Fun and excitement,
Play and wonder,
Exploration, discovery,
Freedom and adventure,
Safety and security,
Growing up, spreading your wings.

Where did they go?...
Can they be found again?
Enjoyed?
Exulted in?

Maybe so.

But first, to mourn, to grieve, to rage, to weep, to cry.
To grieve what has been lost and cannot be regained.

I want to weep with that child,
I want to cry as that child.
I want to be enraged for that child.
I want to protect that child.
I want to embrace my child,
hold him,
comfort him,
nurture him.

I want to exult in life with that little boy,
nurture him,
encourage him,
free him....

Poetry is followed by another new entry that acknowledges the importance of others even in so solitary a pursuit as writing — participation in a *writers' group*.

> "...my writing group. It was the first time in my life I had connected emotionally with anyone, male or female." — Kurt, 39, Georgia

> "VOICES in Action has a SIG (Special Interest Group) writing group. It has been helpful to know that others ALLLL over the country are in the same boat. Being a survivor makes you feel very very very alone (part of my abuse was severe isolation). Knowing that there are others out there helps." — Benn, 32, Georgia

Next in frequency of response is *writing books*.

> "...a lot of my ongoing recovery was through my writing. I think the book has a lot to do with where I am at on many, many levels." — Timothy, 37, Alabama

Other topics related to writing (each receives a single mention) are *correspondence, personal histories, stories, essays*, and even *destroying some writing*.

> "...VOICES...Pen pal groups (SIG)." — Scott, 41, Michigan

> "...writing the story in all its horrible details. Looking and saying what for so long was impossible to see or say." — Michael, 40, New Jersey

> "...my writing kept me going. In one...story, I will kill off the child, because at the time I felt it was the only way that the adult could survive. It would still be a few years before I realised I could still keep part of the child I once was. In fact, I found him to be the strongest part." — Gregory, 37, Ontario, Canada

"I have also found a great deal of healing in the destruction of some [of my writing]...burning, burying, shredding, casting to the river, water-soluble ink in the rain, but never throwing in the garbage." — Keith, 31, Quebec, Canada

Here is an example of the use of symbolic confrontation in mid-recovery. There will be further discussion of *confrontational writing* in the section covering later stage recovery. **Bobby, 31, Georgia,** sent a copy of his letter to an abuser who died before it was written. His accompanying note to me explains its significance:

"...the enclosed letter, which I had written in my journal...I feel it was an important part of my recovery. I've moved even further since I wrote the letter. My recovery is moving along very good. I have so much more understanding about what happened to me now."

Here is Bobby's letter in its entirety:

A Letter to Buck

If you could speak to me from where you are now Buck, I wonder what you would say. Would you say you were sorry for hurting me the way you did? Or would you even care? Would you try and tell me once again that it was all my fault? If you did, it would not work this time. I'm not a helpless child anymore. A child can never be blamed for the actions of an adult, especially when that child had absolutely no control over what that adult was doing to them.

Would you tell me that you still loved me? Am I still your special boy? I did just like you told me to do; I never told anyone about what you were doing to me. No matter how much you made it hurt, I remained silent. I'm not sure if the reason was to protect your memory, or maybe it was to protect my future. I still feel guilty and ashamed for allowing you to do those things to me. I'm mad at myself for believing all the lies you told me. I'm angry that no one ever told me that what you were doing was bad. I'm angry because you taught me all the bad things that can happen to children by doing them to me, instead of someone teaching me what to do if anyone tried exactly what you accomplished doing. I kept all your secrets, and then I grew to an age where I began to wonder if what you were doing was wrong. I fought back and you abandoned me. You left me to try and put the pieces of my life back together alone. I understand now that I'm older why you did this. You were afraid that I would expose you to the world. After all you did, you were nothing more than a coward. So for that reason you stayed away. That still didn't help me to understand what had happened to me during those five years you abused me. I was like a young child lost in the wilderness. Thanks to your training there was no one that I could trust to help me find my way back home again. Even if someone had come to me and offered to show me the way, I would have refused their help. You taught me to fear others, and by example you proved to me that no one could be trusted. I knew if I was ever going to get home again, it would have to be on my own.

Buck, I often wonder if I come to where you are now, what would you do? Would you once again come to me and show me the way? Or would you hide from my presence, ashamed for the pain you caused? You made me into a person I do not know. Do you feel any of the guilt that I feel? I wish I could understand why you hurt me the way you did. Is it true what I've been told? That you never really loved me — I was just your victim. They say that at some point I will have to forgive you. Do you even want forgiveness? You never asked for it. How much of a man did it make you feel like when you took a nine-year-old boy and made him satisfy your sexual desires? Did you feel like an even bigger man when you beat me for not performing to your satisfaction? Remind me when we meet again to show all my gratitude for all you did for me.

◆ ◆ ◆ ◆ ◆

OTHER CREATIVE ACTIVITIES

As with endeavors related to writing, survivors report continuing importance of other activities and creativity, with some change of emphasis. In mid-recovery, a new category is mentioned most frequently — *sports* and *exercise.*

> "...sports. First alone, then team sports. I had a body. I could use it." — Rob, 33, Idaho

> "I ran, but this time I was not running away. I ran for life, for strength, to breathe." — Hector, 58, Mexico

We see renewed commitment to life, health and self care, rediscovered appreciation of one's body, continued desire to interact with others, and discovery of healthier ways to feel good. In addition to sports and exercise, there are new references to related pursuits — *healthy living, nutrition,* and *yoga.*

> "...eating right, getting enough sleep and exercising regularly. Getting myself into shape for a good life." — Blaine, 40, Utah

> "...the practice of Iyengar-style yoga helped me to draw out body memories that remained at a cellular level, and that would otherwise not have been available to me. The experience was at first confusing, and not always pleasant, but it did speed the process." — David, 57, New Mexico

These are followed, in roughly equal numbers, by *art, music,* and *singing.*

> "When I was young, they told me I didn't have any talent. Just another one of their lies. I started drawing and painting. They were wrong. Every child is an artist." — Thor, 55, Washington State

> "I found my voice and began to sing." — Frank, 37, Idaho

There are single mentions of *roller skating, tai chi, baths, hugging, walking, photography,* and taking a *sex education course.* Some men write of using animate or inanimate *objects* to practice caring for others and accepting love; *pets* are mentioned, along with *stuffed animals* and *images from the past.*

> **"...learning to reach out and touch and relate to my dog and, in turn, to allow the dog to love me."** — Michael, 46, North Carolina

> **"Most of all, and this sounds really silly, I found courage from an old picture of myself taken at age five. He was — rather, *I* was — quite a boy."** — Osvaldo, 41, Iowa

TAKING DIFFICULT BUT NECESSARY STEPS

The numbers in this area are down only slightly, but there is almost total change of emphasis. The abuse was realized and acknowledged earlier in recovery; there is no need to do it at this point. Only one survivor now writes of his need to break the silence. During mid-recovery efforts are directed toward *wider disclosure* and greater *honesty.*

> **"...to tell others what had been done to me."** — Matsuo, 21, Japan

> **"...going public. That is, 'telling the truth about my incest experiences *without fear* of the consequences.' *The truth hurts.*"** — Xandu the Giant, 33, New York

> **"...exposing all my secrets to my wife and anyone else who I felt safe with, so I could start to live without secrets and the need for defenses."** — Adrian, 45, Massachusetts

> **"...being honest even when I didn't want to be opened a new world for me. I could hold my head up at last!"** — Aaron, 29, New Mexico

No one writes of the need to *achieve* sobriety or abstinence. With continuing recovery come different needs and emphases. There is now a major increase in the category that includes *continuing to tell or share one's story, public speaking,* and *wider disclosure* in general.

> **"I made my abuse known to certain family and friends."** — John, 61, Maryland

> **"Once I began talking, no one could shut me up."** — Les, 60, New Zealand

> "...speaking publicly and not being ashamed of what had happened to me." — Gordon, 57, New South Wales, Australia

> "Opening up to my sisters also helped tremendously. One sister said, 'God, I thought I was the only one, or I was making it up." — Chris, 22, Texas

In addition, men have begun to acknowledge the risky experiences of *honesty with oneself* as well as others,

> "I stopped pretending. When I stopped trying to fool people into thinking everything was ok, I stopped fooling myself." — Bo, 56, Nebraska

asking for help and support,

> "As my recovery progressed, I became aware of the fact that I could evaluate and ask for support." — Jim, 26, Massachusetts

taking *time off from work,*

> "...admitting that I couldn't do it all. I took a leave from my job and turned my attention to getting better." — Tony, 44, Nevada

confrontation,

> "...for me, confrontation was essential. It broke the silent vow for me to die with the secret. It gave me back my power. It said that I was no longer prepared to be a victim. It released the shame and the guilt, and whether they were prepared to accept it or not, it said that I was no longer going to carry it. And it told me that 'it happened.'" — John, 32, Newfoundland, Canada

avoiding toxic people,

> "...removing myself from the abusive and from the primarily nonsupportive people in my life. As I kept myself removed from them, my life became immediately and tremendously better." — Bob, 48, Illinois

and *setting safe boundaries* — sexual and otherwise.

> **"MOVING was very helpful, start over, start fresh. If the memories overwhelm you — go heal! Go away!...Find a place that your soul is happy. Check out the energy — your heart will know what/where is right." — Benn, 32, Georgia**

ATTENTION TO SELF

At this point we notice the beginning of a trend that will continue strongly throughout the recovery process. Along with his connection (or reconnection) with others, there are profound changes in how the survivor views and treats himself.

> **"...a determination for survival..." — Paul, 43, County Devon, England**

> **"Although it's hard at times, I don't apologise for what was done to me, and the condition it left me in." — Paddy, 49, Queensland, Australia**

> **"...seeing ways I was opening, relaxing, and deepening. I found myself more assured and relaxed with men, willing and able to define boundaries with women." — David, 54, Colorado**

This direction becomes even more pronounced later. In addition to awareness of *inner strength*, mid-recovery responses voice the positive needs of *self-exploration*, *self-appreciation*, *self-affirmation*, and general *self-focus*.

> **"...myself, deep deep down that innate ability to open my eyes to face yet another day and another day...I would be dead Without the resources of inner strength." — Ron, 52, Missouri**

> **"...if I wasn't going to live as a victim, I had to find out who I was." — William, 62, South Carolina**

> **"...Within myself — pride, dignity, and my own self-esteem." — Jim, 24, County Strathclyde, Scotland**

> **"...affirming my basic goodness." — Randy, 36, Tennessee**

> **"...embracing myself and honoring myself and allowing myself time to heal. Recovery is not a contest." — Tom, 40, Michigan**

Men are talking about *commitment* — to themselves and to life, *taking responsibility* for their own lives, *changing their beliefs, reactions, habits,* and *behavior.*

> "I was able to put aside a lifetime preoccupation with suicidal feelings which had led to several serious attempts but had sullied every aspect of my life. I ruled out suicide and made a commitment to live for the first time.." — John, 58, Massachusetts

> "...I said — I will not die as a victim." — Ali, 53, Egypt

> "...realizing that I had to do it for myself. Nobody was going to do it for me." — Will, 55, Arkansas

> "...fighting to believe there is something better for me out there — I'm not defective!" — Aaron, 29, New Mexico

> "Since January 1, I took the resolution of respecting myself by not acting out sexually — by not using myself or others as sex objects. It has been a few months now, and I feel very proud of myself for making this decision. Even though the temptations of acting out are still there, I feel I am important enough to keep respecting myself in this way. I realize that self-respect goes hand in hand with self-esteem." — Daniel, 39, New Brunswick and Ontario, Canada

Frank, 34, New York, gave permission to include this poem of commitment to himself, which he wrote and read at a male survivors' weekend:

> Alone I stand —
> A scary place, too frightening to name;
> A place obscured by darkness,
> Loneliness and shame.
>
> Why stand I here, in this strange place?
> My quest remains the same.
> My boyhood once was taken;
> It's this I must reclaim.

> **This boy in me has hidden well.**
> **It's been too dark to see.**
> **With time, alone I may not stand;**
> **Perhaps I'll stand with me.**

◆ ◆ ◆ ◆ ◆

We are at the start of an exciting new direction, one that will become an impressive groundswell.

ATTENTION TO OTHERS

The changes we witness in the male survivor's attention to himself extend to his concern for others. In mid-recovery, we see emerging interest in *helping victims* and *working with and for other survivors*.

> **"It was important for me to share what I had learned to give back to society some of the good that I had experienced since I started my recovery. I became a volunteer at the...sexual assault center...by speaking on the subject of sexual assault...I was able to make an impact on other people — especially males — as to the seriousness of the problem and the available resources." — Mark, 34, Alberta, Canada**

What we are seeing is not the survivor's pre-recovery attempt to avoid his own issues by paying attention to other people's problems. Instead, there is a feeling of connection, manifested by a desire to *share* with other survivors what he has learned during recovery and a need to *do something worthwhile*. He is *actively taking charge*, accomplishing change in the wider world. This human, *altruistic*, and powerful response will continue and grow even stronger.

> **"...sharing my experience with others..." — Steve, 42, South Dakota**

> **"...being involved with 'the Banner Project' where, with the support of other survivors, male and female, I was able to speak publicly of my abuse and healing journey and the need to break the silence of sexual abuse." — Curt, 43, Wisconsin**

> "...pursuing a proactive stance on recovery, including publishing two self-help books, doing my doctoral dissertation on sexual abuse survivors in ministry, organizing self-help conferences, speaking on the subject before various groups." — Treetop, 40, Arizona

RELIGION AND SPIRITUALITY

As male survivors start looking beyond themselves, they often show greater concern with spirituality and religious *belief* and *practice*. While there is now a slight decline in number of references to *prayer* and *devotions* (which are often solitary pursuits), twice as many men write about *God* or a *Higher Power, religion* or *spirituality, meditation,* and *religious teachings* — both Western and Eastern. These numbers are not huge, but they are growing.

> "God had not abandoned me." — Luis, 35, Colombia

> "...reconnecting with my spirituality, which had long been denied..." — Mark, 34, Alberta, Canada

> "...developing a daily meditation practice...especially helpful and meaningful to me..." — Erik, 47, South Dakota

> "Meditation, or the practice of spirituality, continued to be my strongest ally." — David, 57, New Mexico

> "...Hindu teachings and the *Siddha Yoga* Path." — Eston, 43, Kentucky

> "...my Judaism, prayer, the morning blessings..." — Ira, 44, New York

At a workshop, **Ira, 44, New York,** spoke of his religion (Judaism) and religious practice and its importance in his recovery. During an evening of creativity presentation, he talked about having brought his morning blessings and chants to the workshop, intending to perform them privately. Later he decided to share them with the group, saying that, although they have private meaning for him, **"to do blessings in public with people knowing what it means to**

me — [is] *about my recovery.*" Ira read a traditional *Shabbat* (Sabbath) blessing, first in Hebrew, then in English, adding lines of his own (shown here in italics) that had special meaning for many listeners. Here is some of Ira's blessings:

Blessed is the Eternal our God, Ruler of the universe, who has implanted mind and instinct within every living being.

Blessed is the Eternal our God, who has made me to be free.

Blessed is the Eternal our God, who brings freedom to the captive.

Blessed is the Eternal our God, whose power lifts up the fallen.

Blessed is the Eternal our God, who makes firm each person's steps.

Blessed is the Eternal our God, who gives strength to the weary.

Blessed is the Eternal our God, who removes sleep from the eyes, slumber from the eyelids. (*To awaken the parts of me that have been asleep for many years.*)

Lord our God and God of all ages, school us in Your *Torah* [the Five Books of Moses — the Pentateuch] and bind us to your *Mitzvot* [Blessings].

Help us to keep far from sin, to master temptation, and to avoid falling under its spell. May our darker passions not rule us, nor evil companions lead us astray.

THE ROLE OF FEELINGS

In the middle stages of recovery, the subject of *expressing emotions* remains relatively neglected, unappreciated, or avoided. There is even a slight decrease in the number of direct references to feelings. Beyond the general area of expressing feelings, the only specific emotional activity mentioned is *grieving*.

> **"...space to grieve." — Michael, 28, County Dublin, Ireland**

I wonder whether, after reluctantly allowing themselves to feel the pain of early recovery, male survivors are hoping that the emotional part is over. It's not, but things aren't as messy as they were. As recovery progresses, focus on emotions changes in quantity and quality. Many find it surprising that these changes are not as unpleasant or frightening as they had feared; they are just another part of creating a full, rich, self-realized life.

> "*...paying attention* to my feelings instead of 'medicating' them with drugs, booze, sex, television, food, or music. *Feelings don't kill you.*" — Xandu the Giant, 33, New York

FORGIVENESS, RISK, AND CHANGES

There is still no mention of any form of forgiveness (I find it a healthy sign that survivors are not inclined to give in to external agendas), or much new risk–taking, enjoyment of the present or hope for the future, yet we can recognize seeds of change.

> "...understanding I cannot change my molested childhood any more than I can expect a stone to fall upward, helped me let go the chronic rage which blocked my recovery — not to 'forgive', but to be free of it..." — Lawrence, 62, New York

At this point appears the first mention of *dating* and "*inner child work*."

> "...to start dating again — seeing and spending time with women in a sexual and nonsexual way helped to rebuild my self-esteem." — Mark, 34, Alberta, Canada

> "...reaching for the scared little boy and offering him my hand." — Arthur, 65, Oregon

This is one of two short poems contributed by **Eston, 43, Kentucky**:

Free Child

Crisp and clear as autumn air, his knowledge is there —
   without his knowing.
He begets nothing. Nothing that is showing.
Starting the day in any way that gets the blood a-flowing

He begins to think of reasons in pink
and stars that should stop glowing.

Walk with him a mile or so and do it under stress.
Give to him a seed to grow or give him nothing less.

This is just the start. "You ain't seen nothin' yet."

Part Three

LATE RECOVERY

M y third question addresses the survivor's current situation:

"In support of my recovery today, I focus on..."

The answers to this question, although they all refer to *present time support and activities*, reflect a wide range of individual experience. Some of the male survivors quoted here have been working steadily at their recovery for many years; others are relatively new to the process. Despite these differences, I refer to the responses to this question as representing the *later stages of recovery*, compared with *early healing* and *mid-stage recovery*. I hope you will find it helpful to learn about resources that are valued currently by other male survivors.

> **"There are now entire days when I do not think of myself as a victim. This is a wonder beyond measure." — Ali, 53, Egypt**

> **"It often seems that today...is the real difficult part of my healing, in that I now have to use what I have learned!" — John, 32, Newfoundland, Canada**

In addition, I hope that it will be as obvious to you as it is to me that the differences in responses to the three questions demonstrate a pattern of genuine progress in recovery. That is, RECOVERY IS REAL, IT IS POSSIBLE, AND IT MATTERS! I find evidence of these truths everywhere I go. The work done by survivors pays off. The dividends are enormous. And everyone shares in the benefits.

Let's take a look at some of these changes.

BOOKS AND READING

By late recovery, there is a dramatic drop in the number of responses concerning *books* and *reading*. As their lives continue to blossom, male survivors become less dependent upon those resources. Far fewer individuals make nonspecific reference to books, reading, and learning. No book receives more than a single mention. It appears that once this degree of recovery has been attained, and survivors have begun to *thrive*, reading becomes one activity among many — a source of enjoyment and/or information, rather than a lifeline.

> **"...keeping up with current research & literature..."** — **Roger, 44, Florida**

> **"...the pure pleasure of poetry."** — **Joel, 34, Connecticut**

Some books are touchstones, trusted reminders of progress.

> **"I read it [*Victims No Longer*] every night before I go to sleep and it's like a friend to me. It gives me comfort and hope and strength and new ideas and lets me feel I'm not alone."** — **Scott, 43, Brazil**

Survivors have incorporated what they learned from their studies and are moving on with their lives.

The eight★ books and authors cited in response to Question 3 are about equally divided between familiar and new ones. They are:

The Courage to Heal by Ellen Bass and Laura Davis

Come Here by Richard Berendzen

Lead Us Not into Temptation by Jason Berry

Half the House by Richard Hoffman

Abused Boys by Mic Hunter

Speaking Our Truth by Neal King

Facing the Fire by John H. Lee

Victims No Longer by Mike Lew

Alice Miller (no specific work mentioned)

★ Once again, you may have counted more than eight items on this list. This time it is because someone cites *Come Here* as having been written by Jason Berry. I decided to list both *Come Here* (written by Richard Berendzen) and Jason Berry's relevant work (*Lead Us Not into Temptation*).

Several men state that *Internet/World Wide Web/On-Line* services continue to be important to them, but even in cyberspace there is a significant shift of emphasis.

> "...continued involvement with others who need support and healing. I am no longer Section Leader of IWA (I Was Abused forum on CompuServe), but am now Section Leader of a new section called 'Loving a Survivor' (LAS) ...open to people who are in a relationship with a survivor of abuse and is designed to give them support and help them learn how to help the survivor(s) in their life." — Doug, 33, California

> "...and continued involvement with the Usenet news groups that I have found so helpful." — Warren, 31, Ontario, Canada

SAFE ENVIRONMENTS

By late recovery, a reasonable sense of safety has been established. The total number of references to safe environments drops considerably, and the type of refuge changes completely. There is no mention of hospitals, residential treatment centers, or rehabilitation programs. There no longer are any nonspecific allusions to "safe places." In fact, the only acknowledgment of environment is reference to *nature* and the *outdoors*.

> "...regular activity that touches my soul...spending time in nature, especially any time in the wilderness, such as canoe trips..." — Erik, 47, South Dakota

> "...hanging out at the Coast, rock climbing, lakes, mountains, old growth forests." — Clay, 24, Oregon

Although it is always wise to protect oneself from real danger, by late recovery, the male survivor has developed a sense of a more benign world — a place of both dangers and safety. Much of his sense of safety is an outgrowth of the healing process. He has gained a surer understanding of how to determine which people and situations are relatively safe, and which are more dangerous. He has learned to establish and maintain reasonable boundaries, and therefore no longer needs to hide away from life.

> "I know that I have much work still to do in my therapy and my living. Both improve." — Ryszard, 22, Poland

> "...living my life! I actually look forward to leaving the house." — Arthur, 65, Oregon

PROFESSIONAL RESOURCES

In late recovery, the importance of *professional therapy or counseling* decreases greatly. Although significant numbers of men still acknowledge the value of some form of ongoing therapy, it no longer occupies the same degree of centrality — and the emphasis continues to change and grow. This is true of both individual and group work.

> "...continuing spiritual development and psychotherapy that focuses on the development of self and self in relation to others." — Doug, 57, California

> "...now the therapy reminds me of the many changes that I have made in my life." — Peter, 43, South Africa

The number of men citing *individual counseling* or *therapy* remains about the same at all three stages of recovery. However, as recovery progresses, there is a dramatic drop in references to the individual *counselor* or *therapist* (More than ten times as many men cite their individual therapist in early compared to late recovery — and over eight times as many in mid-stage as in late).

Late recovery participation in *therapy groups* is still about a third greater than during early healing, but has dropped in importance by well over half from the middle stages. This late-stage decrease occurs across the board — in general or nonspecified group therapy, mixed gender survivor groups, general men's groups, and male survivor groups. However, for many men, the right group still makes all the difference.

> "...finding a group of male survivors to mourn the loss of childhood and rid myself of leftover ghosts." — Gene, 32, California

> "SIA meetings, group therapy (all male survivors), and a support group of friends are the key elements." — Tom, 36, New York

> "The group...challenges me to affirmative thinking and the setting of boundaries." — George, 61, Washington State

> "It took me over sixty phone calls to find the group I wanted. None came upon a closed door—each person gave me two to five references. Eventually, I found it, and, in retrospect, even the searching itself was healthy.... I owe my life as it is right now to my Wednesday men's group. Without their love and support, I would be in dire shape. Any issue that concerns me in my life this week is appropriate for discussion here, and there is no judgment passed or verdict rendered...just pure love laid upon me for who I am." — Keith, 31, Quebec, Canada

This trend is confirmed in the area of one time events. There are half the number of references to *workshops and retreats* in late recovery as in the early stages. Over five times as many men include workshops and retreats in their response to Question 2 as compared to Question 3. But for a significant number of survivors the importance of such events continues unabated.

> "My favorite retreat center is 700 km (400 miles) away, and worth every step. Things are opened in an intense weekend that are impossible to touch in that single hour per week of therapy." — Keith, 31, Quebec, Canada

> "Here I am, still surviving...my mind and body still quiver with excitement, energy, emotions of every color, size, shape, and description. I consider that a success. Yea!... I believe I've shed a great deal of shame this weekend. After coming out years ago, the least I owe myself is the same level of pride and accomplishment in dealing with my recovery." — Clain, 38, New York [written after a weekend workshop]

> "...was great for me. More is still unfolding and is helping me to pull together the years of work I've done regarding the sexual abuse I've experienced. Being with other male survivors was the most healing aspect of the weekend — I've followed up with some of the men...following the weekend my work is taking a different direction. I have a

clearer perspective, which is enabling me to assert myself more truly with family and friends." — Rick, 41, New Jersey [written after a weekend workshop]

Now there are no references to conferences, educational seminars, or academic courses. Perhaps, by late recovery, life is being *lived*, not studied.

"...to experience what I had only read of." — Julian, 30, Hong Kong

"...attending to 'building a life' as a method of recovery, rather than completing recovery in order to 'have a life.'" — Erik, 47, South Dakota

Accompanying the movement away from professional and organized resources is a dramatic drop (of over 60 percent) in the importance of peer organizations compared to the earlier stages of recovery. The most frequently cited program continues to be *SIA/ISA* (Survivors of Incest Anonymous/Incest Survivors Anonymous).

"I still check in regularly with other members (of ISA). It gives me hope and perspective." — Thor, 55, Washington State

There are some nonspecific references to *twelve-step programs and principles* and a couple of mentions of *ACA/ACOA* (Adult Children of Alcoholics) groups. Beyond those, there is only one mention each of *AA* (Alcoholics Anonymous), *SLAA* (Sex and Love Addicts Anonymous), *Reevaluation Counseling*, and *Moving Forward*.

"...taking one day at a time; keeping involved with people." — Bob, 39, Pennsylvania

"I fellowship with other 'Adult Children' (ACOA) as a safe place for me to share feelings, real emotional stuff that matters, for I matter!" — Mark, 34, West Virginia

"...continuing to attend AA and SIA meetings keeps me focused and cognizant of where I have been and where I am headed..." — John, 32, Newfoundland, Canada

It looks as though "moving forward" has come to mean moving away from a specific recovery focus in the direction of more complete embracing of life.

SAFE AND SUPPORTIVE PERSONS

"Where paths that have affinity for each other intersect, the whole world looks like home." — Hermann Hesse

As the male survivor's self-esteem grows and healthy self-reliance blooms — as comfort with his life increases — as the compartments open up and he continues moving toward a more fully integrated life — dependence upon a limited number of safe individuals wanes. As occurred with professionals and peer organizations, there is a sharp decline in the category of *safe and supportive persons*. This decrease doesn't mean that the male survivor no longer needs people as touchstones in his life. It certainly doesn't mean that all people are equally safe and supportive. There is always going to be the need for important *friends*, family members, partners, and other special people to whom he can turn when things get rough, but by late recovery, survivors recognize that there are many good, safe people in the world.

"...those around me that I care about..." — David, 35, Wyoming

"...a close circle of friends who know..." — Geoff, 35, Pennsylvania

"...my true friends. — J.V., 28, Kenya

It is no longer just your individual therapist, a single author, your partner, spouse, or a few fellow survivors who can understand what you're going through and offer a hand to grasp — a shoulder to lean on. The number of safe, supportive people in the world is far greater than you had ever imagined. The world is a better place than you had dreamed. Some survivors, recognizing that they were lied to about many other things, go back to *investigate* the truths and lies about their own families. This new information can provide new and surprising *allies*.

"My mother kept me isolated from other family members. She was quite successful.... I knew near to nothing of my family history. Now I have started to investigate. The investigation increases my understanding of my own background." — Hamid, 52, Denmark

"...my Aunt F___. She was the first one in my family who told me the truth about my childhood. She is someone I can always count on." — Jimmy, 23, Mississippi

◆ ◆ ◆ ◆ ◆

My intent in distributing the Request for Resources was to elicit information from *male* survivors. I received the following response from a woman in Canada who had something important to say, so she ignored my instructions. For that, I am grateful. It is important to acknowledge our allies. In the midst of the attention that is finally being paid to the serious subject of female abusers, we must recognize the importance of protective and understanding women — of loving and dedicated mothers. We need to be reminded that some people do understand. We need to remember that a person doesn't have to be perfect or have all the answers in order to be an important ally. Being open, nondefensive. and caring makes all the difference. Thank you, Kay, your statement is a fine reminder.

An Ally's Statement

I am a mother of a sexually abused boy. Initially it was difficult as little information was available about sexually abused boys. There were no counselling programs that dealt with young boys as victims of sexual abuse. Our support has been bibliotherapy. Books have been a great resource for us. A book is handy in a crisis when no one is available to comfort and give support. The words of other survivors or the author comfort. If issues or flashbacks come up, the books are right there to give understanding and suggestions on how to deal with the situation. The first book that was available to us was *Victims No Longer*. I found some hope in my attempt to offer support and understanding for my son. I have read most of the books and articles about boys and men who have been sexually abused. I have read aloud and shared the information so that he would not feel so alone and estranged from the rest of the world — having been sexually abused. I have also encouraged him to read the books.

There is a stigma around male survivors of sexual abuse. A stigma that I don't think exists for female survivors. The stigma is that if a boy or male reveals he has been sexually abused, society tends automatically to presume that he is going to become a perpetrator. In a relationship between a man and a woman, the man who has been sexually abused as a child is more vulnerable to the suspicion of being an abuser. This could be due to our socially acceptable belief that men are perpetrators. Women are not seen as perpetrators. This stigma has had great impact on recovery as it makes it difficult to talk about abuse.

There is a belief in society that men cannot be raped. I have heard men and women say so. When a man who has been sexually abused is in a relationship with a woman and she doesn't believe men can be raped, it hurts. It hurts the intimacy of the relationship and creates men with masks. For that man it is like a second rape — by not being believed by friends, [the] justice system, and society as a whole. Sexually abused men need support and nurturing just like female survivors.

These are some of the realities that sexually abused boys and men have to confront today. Books and education of society will, I hope, change all this. I have read John Andrews's book *Not Like Dad* [see the Resource Bibliography] and it has been an inspiration for all of us. John Andrews's personal struggles through the recovery process are encouraging and have given me strength to keep fighting for services for male survivors of sexual abuse. It has been lonely many times trying to deal with the pain and anger of sexual abuse.

I think it is important to deal with the guilt over sexual arousal during the abuse. I have explained erection as a reflex. The erection reflex is stimulated as a result of touch — not because they wanted to have an erection. It is just like when a doctor hits the right spot on your knee. It stretches out and there is nothing you can do to prevent it. Erection is partly a reflex and happens because of reaction to touch.

One of the hardest issues has been the anger toward me. The anger is appropriate, as he feels I was not there to protect him from the abuse. This anger has to be dealt with and it is important to justify that anger toward women, then work through the anger in a constructive way. If the anger is not dealt with, boys and men may misplace it onto innocent women. I intellectually understand the anger, but emotionally it is difficult to deal with.

There are times when a word of caution is in place toward counsellors and other helping professionals. There are support staff who — in the initial stage of treatment — ask for details to verify the sexual abuse. I call this covert voyeurism, where they satisfy their own sexual curiosity and needs with details of the abuse. Why does the family of the survivor have to confirm the abuse with details? I have refused to return because of that. The most helpful response when a survivor or family member talks about sexual abuse is, "I am sorry to hear that — it must have been painful. What can I do to help you today?"

— Kay, 43, British Columbia, Canada

Although the numbers are far smaller than in the middle stage, *friend(s)* continues to be the category of safe persons most frequently singled out during late recovery.

"...loving friends in the present." — Alford, 55, Minnesota

"...letting more of my friends learn my secrets and care for me." — Mohammed, 42, Pakistan

"My friends take me for who I am and let me know that I am worthy of love." — Rod, 48, Rhode Island

Second place is still occupied by *spouse/partner/lover/primary other.*

"... trusting my experience and being in a good, supportive relationship with my wife." — Moe, 63, Massachusetts

"...my lover. He is also my best friend." — Rob, 33, Idaho

But there is about equally frequent mention of various kinds of *body workers* (a significant increase),

> "...deep structural body work..." — Lloyd, 44, New York

> "...integration of physical therapies. It surprises me that now I can let my body be touched." — Alejandro, 27, Argentina

> "This has been very helpful, in releasing memories and trauma locked up in my body." — Murray, 41, Ontario, Canada

and *caring community* or *support network* (an even larger increase).

> "...developing a secure network of allies." — Jim, 42, New Hampshire

> "...community. I am blessed with so many good people around me." — William, 62, South Carolina

> "...building a support network through increased social interaction..." — Warren, 31, Ontario, Canada

All these responses provide mounting evidence that the survivor's world continues to expand.

While there is a jump in the number of responses mentioning *children*, there is a fairly large decline overall in the category of *family* or *family member(s)*.

> "...my kids, who love me and remind me that I can make a difference." — Bo, 56, Nebraska

> "...and my little granddaughter brings sunshine. She is a happy child...reminds me that the abuse in my family has ended." — Juan, 67, Spain

> "I have a sister who has consistently been extremely supportive. I could not have done it without her." — Murray, 41, Ontario, Canada

A few men write about unspecified *supportive person(s)*, and there are single mentions of *colleagues* and *chosen family*.

> "...the support I get from a lot of people." — Blaine, 40, Utah

> "...my loving relationships, those who I consider family —
> biological and otherwise — and I focus on the many ways
> I can enrich others, while FINALLY allowing others to
> enrich my life." — Osvaldo, 41, Iowa

Finally, there is a huge decline in references to *other survivors*, whether male, female, or of unspecified gender. Late recovery brings fewer than half as many such mentions as early healing, and less than a third compared with mid-stage recovery. At this later stage, only one individual includes the category of *hearing other survivors' stories*. But, while it is large, this change is not universal.

> "I always enjoy sharing my healing path with other male
> survivors. Finding new friends along the path to recov-
> ery helps me mark my way." — Scott, 41, Michigan

> "...male and female survivors are allies in the twin causes
> of recovery and changing the world." — Murray, 41,
> Ontario

> "...where I live,...here in the mountains, three days ago
> ...we held my first survivors' meeting in my room. Then,
> afterward, we held an SLAA meeting (DASA we call it in
> Brazil)." — Scott, 43, Brazil

From talking with male survivors in late recovery, and from the tone of their written responses, I am convinced that the trend we see here does not represent a return to isolation. Rather, it is one result of living a more expansive and better integrated life — producing greater varieties of interaction with larger numbers of people.

> "I choose when to spend time with friends and when I
> would rather be alone. I like to be with people and I like
> being with myself." — Stefan, 51, South Africa

> "Now when I travel I talk to strangers. I make new
> friends. I accept people for who they are." — Terry, 49,
> Tennessee

> "...that more people have entered my life. It is because I
> let them be close to me." — Ismail, 40, Malaysia

There is redirection of attention — away from activities that are purely related to abuse recovery — toward greater diversity of interests. The *recovered* survivor is living more richly. His life is not problem-free, but now it encompasses far more than his difficulties.

WRITING ACTIVITIES

For male survivors the importance of *writing* remains constant throughout the recovery process.

> "Writing and publishing my story helps in the strangest ways. While it was (and remains) extremely cathartic, it also challenges me to be a survivor and fight back for the life that I was always meant to have. Today I have to challenge my 'victimhood' and create healthier ways to define me as a man and as a person. For years, I defined myself by my ability to drink and party. Then I found pride in my ability to work and produce. Early in recovery, it was as if [I] collapsed into being a victim, permitting myself not to have to explain, apologize for, or challenge my dysfunctions. Now, if I am to continue to heal and grow, I have to tell myself that enough has been taken — I will give no more." — John, 32, Newfoundland, Canada

There is a slight increase in the number of people listing *nonspecific writing, journaling,* or *keeping a log.*

> "Today I still focus on my writing, as it has been my strongest weapon in my recovery." — Gregory, 37, Ontario, Canada

> "...my writing is clearer and stronger..." — Teishiro, 34, Japan

> "...journaling every day, taking time for me." — Charles, 45, Illinois

> "...me and my thoughts. I am now doing...a thirty-day thinking log. I *honestly* log any sexual thinking that I have for thirty days, then bring it in to my therapist and group, then read it to them and get feedback." — Rodger, 31, Montana

In keeping with an overall increase in references to confrontation (which will be discussed later), there is more *confrontational writing*.

> **"In therapy my focus has been on confronting my perpetrator and I have just written a letter to him." — Doug, 33, California**

During the creativity portion of a weekend male survivors' workshop, **Chris, 57, Ohio,** received a standing ovation for his statement that contradicts old negative, shaming messages from his mother. Everyone can identify with some part of Chris's poem; he introduced it this way:

> **"As I listen this morning, the more Peggy keeps coming to the front of my mind. I wonder about that poor soul. Why did I come to her as such a disappointment? What gave her her perception of what men should be — of what her son should be?**
>
> **She spent her life as a mother trying to fix her broken son. She had been cheated by God because He gave her a less than six-foot-tall, athletic, HE MAN son.**
>
> **There are no words to describe how I feel. I tried sooo very hard all my life — all of her life — to be what she wanted and I could not do that!**
>
> **What a shame she did that to me, and what a shame I even tried to fit her twisted model of what a son should be. How wonderful it could have been for us all just to be ourselves.**
>
> **Instead, Peggy, you left me a legacy of never being sure of my own self and a gut-level awareness that I just am not OK."**

Well Let Me Tell You, Peggy:

It's OK to be short
It's OK not to be athletic
It's OK to go to college
It's OK to be gay
It's OK to be tired of working
It's OK to learn to fly an airplane
It's OK to love classical music
It's OK to hate broccoli

It's OK to cry
It's OK to want to be held
It's OK to want to be loved
It's OK to want to be made love to
It's OK to never again say a Hail Mary
It's OK to buy a boat
It's OK to sit on my ass all weekend
It's OK to masturbate
It's OK to lose weight
It's OK to be alone
It's OK not to be in charge
It's OK not to know what I want
It's OK to live near where I grew up
It's OK to let go of the demons
It's OK not to have a career identity
It's OK to cry (I know I said that before)
It's OK not to talk
It's OK to be pissed at God
It's OK to be afraid of the cops
It's OK to be an incest survivor
It's OK to want to live in New Jersey
It's OK to have never said "I Love You" to my parents
It's OK to be scared
It's OK to dislike my job even when thousands are unemployed
It's OK to sleep with stuffed animals

DAMNIT PEGGY — I'M OK! ! ! ! !

For those who continue to maintain journals and logs, the activity appears to have become less central in frequency and intensity, geared more toward *evaluating progress.*

> "I keep a journal infrequently. I do not write in it every day, but on days that I can't stop thinking about the molestation and abuse.... Sometimes they are just blurbs; other times they are lengthy." — Chris, 22, Texas

> "Today I continue to focus on daily journaling. I would say my journal — along with the weekly meetings and my candid correspondence with other male survivors — has been my major means of healing. In my journal I also

> record my dreams and pay close attention to their messages. They have been a remarkably clear indicator confirming the dynamics of the sexual abuse incidents and often are a good indicator of the stage of healing I may be experiencing." — Kristian, 52, Saskatchewan, Canada

The current focus is much more one of *personal creativity* with an added dimension of *disseminating information*. It is consistent with the trends we have observed of male survivors reclaiming their creativity, reaching beyond themselves, and helping others — making the world a better, safer place. Thus, writing *poetry* continues to receive attention, along with *music composition*, writing *letters*, *essays*, *articles*, and a *book*.

> "...going back to *writing* poems and essays about abuse and my recovery *process*. Writing is a path forward for me." — Frederick, 54, Michigan

> "...my music. I teamed up with a local writer who is putting words to my music, and we've even performed locally. Maybe I'll try to write my own words." — Matt, 20, Iowa

> "Exchanging letters with the friends I have met in my traveling connects me with the larger world." — Kemal, 48, Turkey

> "...writing this letter is a big thing for me..." — Bill, 45, Delaware

> "I also write articles on sexual child abuse for the publication *Moving Forward: A Newsjournal for Survivors of Sexual Child Abuse and Those Who Care for Them*. I have...begun a personal book project about being an African-American male survivor. I hope it will help begin to fill an informational void that currently exists in the resources available to those of us living with the effects of sexual child abuse." — Paul, 34, Washington, D.C.

OTHER CREATIVE ACTIVITIES

In addition to the steady importance of writing, there is an explosion of all kinds of creative activity. For some men, *artistic* endeavors provide additional tools for recovery work. For others, newly flowering *creativity* is evidence of their progress.

> **"...positive ways to channel my rage, mostly through artistic expression." — Kurt, 39, Georgia**

> **"...writing and other expressions of my creativity...The abuse, and my subsequent [professional] training, both worked to keep my creativity at a distance. Creative projects — dance, art, sewing, theater, sports, etc. — are valuable emotional outlets. I was very closed off emotionally. Now I know that I need to maintain an emotional connection to the people and the events that are part of day-to-day life. Right now, focusing on theater art is helping me to do that. And besides, it's fun!" — Paul, 34, Washington, D.C.**

◆ ◆ ◆ ◆ ◆

Recovering survivors open up in many ways. As old wounds heal, previously blocked areas of insight, understanding, and creativity begin to flow and flourish. I am reminded of this magic again and again at male survivor workshops when participants share the fruits of their creativity. Here is one example, a skit in the form of a monologue, presented by a male survivor during a weekend workshop. It offers understanding of how all aspects of recovery and liberation struggles are linked — in this example, AIDS support work and abuse recovery. There were few dry eyes in the room when Clain told this story:

The Other Crisis

The following is a recounting of my experience, which contributes to my continuing recovery from childhood abuse.

When my memories began to awaken, I was a volunteer team leader for a group of "Buddies," that is, people who had chosen to become carepartners for People with AIDS. You might say a caregiver to caregivers.

It was a time of witnessing friends, both old and new, growing ill and dying. As further background, I give you a sample of my half of a few telephone conversations with my

coleader Steven. We both are at our daily jobs (as a lawyer and accountant) discussing our team and clients.

Hi, Steve. What's new? Oh, well, Jonathan's client Jerry has been on a Death watch for three weeks now, but, yeah, guess what? Jerry pulled out of it, he's conscious again. Great, huh? So, listen. Jonathan and Sally, you know, the candy striper, right, are planning to sneak Jerry's little dog into his room. Great, huh? I hope they get away with it, too. No, let's not tell the agency.

How's Tom's client? What? A new treatment...Compound Q? Never heard of it. A Chinese cucumber root. Well, as long as Tom's client is very optimistic, well great, let's hope it works. Yea, right, "Q" for Queer. Good for Tom.

Audrey? She had a fight with Bob's day nurse because the nurse actually humiliated Bob for losing control of his bowels in bed again. Well, we're getting a new nurse assigned, but it may take a week. So this nurse stays until replacement. Get this. Audrey told Bob she would bring him prunes just to spite the nurse. Talk about empowerment. Right on, Audrey....

★ ★ ★ ★ ★

Hi, Steve..yeah, Jerry's worse again, Jonathan is working out of town and he's really burned out — toast. He's officially relieved. I'm on it now; it can't be too much longer. What? Oh, well...I..uh..wipe his forehead when he sweats, use those lemon swabs on his lips when they get too dry, squeeze his hand...you know there's not much else... I go every day, after work, sometimes at lunch. I take a cab — the hospital's downtown. No, I'm OK — really it's all right. Jerry deserves this. I'm also doing this for Jonathan, too. I know. Thanks...What? Scott's blind in both eyes now?...horrible. And what? His roommate left. Great — you know that leaves you....Scott's going to be relying on you more and more. Yea, I know you can handle it, but it's...OK, you're OK, I got it.

Audrey took Bob's death pretty well — a real trooper for a new volunteer. Huh? Give her two weeks off and we'll assign her to a new client. Yeah, I heard about the waiting list....

★ ★ ★ ★ ★

My secretary buzzes me to say my mother is on the phone.... *Who? My mother is dead. Oh, wait, I'll take it.*

Marge, you know you are not my mother, please don't...What?
Calm down...my father...a stroke...quadruple bypass...What? Where?
ok, ok, I'll be there. I'm on my way.

After I hang up a wave of nausea comes up. I swallow to keep it down. It returns. Again I swallow. My hands shake violently and I am deeply afraid, frightened.

I pick up the phone to call Darren at crisis management.

Hello, please give me Darren. My name is Clain. Clain, spelled C-L-A-I-N, team leader from team number 3, Manhattan. Get him on the phone. Yes, I am upset. Listen, you're new. You're working in a crisis center, get used to this. Thanks.

Hello, Darren. Listen, I just broke in your new receptionist. Look, I'm in trouble. My father is facing open heart surgery and I'm falling apart here. I've got a lot of bad memories rising up like a backed-up sewer. I need help. No, professional help — big-time. Can you refer me to someone — someone good? What? Thanks. How sweet. I'm touched — really. I'm moved, but I need help. I'm in pain. No, the team is fine. Steven and I are OK — that's not a concern at the moment....

So started the return of horrifying childhood memories and, more importantly, my turning my caregiving skills upon myself. A year later I stepped back from my volunteer work to continue healing my own soul. It's taken three years to get this far. I suppose I have learned more surviving skills than I ever could imagine. I really have needed them.

— Clain, 38, New York

In late recovery this category of *creativity and other life-focused activities* is about twice as large as ever before.

Art remains the most popular activity,

> "...sometimes drawing..." — Svein, 60, Norway

> "I'm taking a life drawing class...to see the beauty of the human body." — David, 27, Oregon

followed by increased interest in *nutrition* and *healthy living*.

> "...on *me*. Gym three to four days a week with a private trainer really helps with loving your body. All relationships

> are better now that I take care of myself." — Gary, 32, New York

> "...overall healthy living." — Ted, 26, Michigan

> "...maintaining my physical health is also important; it keeps me grounded and in my body; it forces me to stay in touch with all aspects of myself..." — Mark, 34, Alberta, Canada

Equally important are *dance, movement,* and a newly discovered interest in *play.*

> "...dancing. Sometimes alone, more and more often with a partner." — Frank, 37, Idaho

> "I dance my life, my happiness, my hopes, my dreams." — Wim, 28, Netherlands

> "...avoiding overwork, underplay, and compulsions..." — Erik, 47, South Dakota

> "Playing with my kids is teaching me a lot." — Van, 41, Colorado

In addition to several *general* references to *creativity,* we see continued interest in *sports* and *exercise,* and renewed interest in *work* and *career.*

> "...plenty of exercise..." — Geoff, 35, Pennsylvania

> "...keeping my body strong and healthy by taking exercise. I play football. It brings me closer with other men and I feel better." — Luis, 22, Costa Rica

> "...positive and productive and creative work I can do." — Phillip, 48, Kentucky

> "My work now helps me be functional and 'act as if' on days when I really want to be a victim. Returning to work was difficult, but essential, in that it forced me to go forward with my life. It is one part of who I am today — no less, no more." — John, 32, Newfoundland, Canada

> "...starting *new* career and *new* relationships." — Paul, 41, New York

Music remains an important interest, listening to it and making it.

"Today I find help from within myself. Music helps me locate hidden feelings, to explore the pain of the past and also come to terms with it. I feel that contemporary composers often bring remarkable insights (perhaps from their own experiences — Richard Marx had a lot to say)." — John, 43, County Mid Glamorgan, Wales

"I still play on my flute for hours on end. Recently, I have let a few close friends hear my music." — Ramesh, 40, India

There are single mentions of *yoga, acting, hobbies, sewing, breathing, massage, unspecified activities, solitude,* and *"enjoyable activities."*

"...yoga and meditation. I am learning a phenomenal amount about myself and life in general through these daily practices, which facilitate acceptance of what is. I am slowly learning to break the three injunctions (don't think, don't talk, don't feel) and am moving toward reaching out to support others in this struggle." — John, 49, Massachusetts

"...a healthy dose of joyful events, along with recovery in moderation." — Scott, 41, Michigan

Finally, *stuffed animals* turn up once again.

"I'm taking care of me, in all stages of my development. The teddy bear I just bought is for the infant who didn't have someone who was soft, warm, and cuddly. And the teddy bear won't screw me in any way." — Oliver, 53, Massachusetts

More and more *freedom* to explore takes the male survivor to wonderful *new places, activities,* and *people.*

"...the freedom of choice. I have to put my time, energy, hope, and love wherever *I* want to." — Tom, 40, Michigan

"...continued spiritual growth, increasing freedom, and more moments of joy." — Mitch, 40, Virginia

"I want to see the World!" — Jürgen, 36, Germany

"...my greater confidence meeting new people." — Matsuo, 21, Japan

> *"...doing things I had never done before!"* — Avoor, 48, Wisconsin

TAKING DIFFICULT BUT NECESSARY STEPS

As might be expected, a benefit of heightened self-esteem and self-confidence is the survivor's greater ability and willingness to take *risks*.

> *"I am willing to be wrong, risk. I have a humor; I even laugh and sometimes joke about myself."* — Bill, 45, Delaware
>
> *"...revealing my vulnerability and needs to my buddies in our survivors' group and to my wife..."* — David, 54, Colorado
>
> *"...I am daring in ways that had been inconceivable."* — Klaus, 56, Switzerland

During this time of late recovery, men are *consolidating* their *gains*.

> *"...reclaiming childhood..."* — Fred, 38, Virginia
>
> *"...building on my past successes. I take affirmation today. I allow my creativity to flow more freely. I play and play and play. I'm twenty months sober as of the seventeenth of this month. I've learned to be more gentle with myself and that I can and do make mistakes and laugh more about this."* — Gug, 46, Pennsylvania

In addition to overall growth of this category, there is impressive change in the specific steps that men consider important. By now, initial acknowledgment of the abuse and the bulk of disclosure have been completed. Increasingly, breaking of secrecy and silence is being directed toward the larger world.

> *"I continue to acknowledge my family history. I have promised myself to write more about it. It certainly gives relief from a considerable amount of emotional grief and pain."* — Clain, 38, New York
>
> *"...bringing out in the open what had been kept a secret for so long, no matter how uncomfortable it makes others feel."* — Michael, 40, New Jersey

In late recovery, the largest single category of response is directed in some way to the scary experience of *giving up control* and *letting himself off the hook*. This vital endeavor is extremely difficult for most male survivors.

> "...giving up the survivor defenses, which are no longer useful." — Chuck, 53, Pennsylvania

> "I survived with an aggressive and combative nature, solely independent. Today, I try to improve on my character flaws and seek help and aid when I need it. I try not to isolate and I let myself participate and feel my natural emotions." — John, 61, Maryland

> "...to 'go with the flow.' I learned this phrase years ago in California. Today it has personal meaning." — Max, 50, Netherlands

> "...no more blaming myself." — Sam, 31, Nigeria

> "...trying to let be what is — and loving myself in the middle of it." — Barrett, 40, New Jersey

> "...living a balanced life. I have learned that it is not selfish to take excellent care of myself and to let others do the same as they choose. To ask directly for what I need, rather than feel a need to control, is vital." — Jim, 26, Massachusetts.

The next largest category covers various forms of *connecting* and *communicating*, *telling* or *sharing their stories*, and *public speaking*.

> "...connecting with other survivors and building a support network and looking after myself." — Mik, 40, Grand Cayman, British West Indies

> "...maintaining the connexions I have established." — Thomas, 45, Germany

> "...communication with my sexual partner." — Bob, 45, California

> "...staying in touch with other male survivors and sharing my present struggles, discouragements and successes..." — Erik, 47, South Dakota

"I make sure that I always discuss my feelings with my wife or a close friend, so that I do not fall back into the habit of suppressing my feelings. By being open and communicative with those closest to me, I avoid letting stress build up in my life." — Mark, 34, Alberta, Canada

"When I meet people I trust totally, I now find it quite easy (to) talk about the past and how it has all affected me. Because now I have lost all the guilt I used to suffer from, it has become much easier to be open about the subject. The more people know and understand the effects child abuse has on people, the better. This fact has a major contribution to self-healing. It is not sympathy that the sufferer seeks, but understanding." — Michael, 43, Surrey, England

"Whenever I make a speech someone always comes up to me afterward to tell me that I was speaking for him, too." — Pat, 42, Nebraska

The survivor now places a greater value on *honesty* — with himself and others.

"...connecting with myself and others in clear, direct, honest ways." — Colin, 33, California

"...being honest and open. I know that I can accept and understand the people I have in my life now, without accepting any of their denial or other dysfunctional behavior. I also frequently remind myself that God is loving and I am, too." — Bob, 48, Illinois

Asking for help and support increases in importance, along with renewed attention to *sobriety* and *abstinence*.

"...asking for the support I need. I have discovered that my friends really do want to help." — Tony, 44, Nevada

"...my own sex and love addiction... Sobriety gives me the clarity to feel my way around inside rather than think." — Paul, 36, Pennsylvania

"...Sobriety!! That and a more spiritual way of life are the tools that help me continue to recover and thrive." — Brad, 35, British Columbia, Canada

CONFRONTATION

There are a growing number of references to *confrontation* — *direct* or *indirect*, *symbolic*, or through the *legal system.*

> **"...telling my story whenever and wherever I can, including confronting my perpetrators..." — Bob, 43, California**

> **"My journey since Kirkridge has been incredible — that is, incredibly frightening, eye-opening, painful at times, and exactly what it's supposed to have been. In a nutshell, I did some very intense regression work, albeit unplanned, and found myself telling my first abuser that I was going to tell — tell everyone what he'd attempted. Mike, it's hard to explain the feelings that I had once I heard my own voice and truly *felt* what I had said. In a very real sense, I took back my own power. Coincidentally, a few days after that session, I ran into that very abuser, someone I have not seen in many years. I was able to draw on the strength of my journey, and knew that he was not going to hurt me anymore." — Frank, 28, Virginia**

> **"...a big step for me...was taking my offender to court. This process has been so empowering for me. I realize that I can never have back what was stolen, but saying, 'You took this from me,' and challenging his actions in a court of law, has given me great strength. This course of action is not for everyone...but for me it has provided a great deal of closure." — Mark, 34, Alberta, Canada**

It cannot be stressed often enough that legal action is something that must be considered very carefully — such actions are not to be undertaken lightly or impulsively. Unless done responsibly and with great care, there is too much potential for retraumatizing.

◆ ◆ ◆ ◆ ◆

An example of the power of confrontation is the following letter from a male survivor to someone who abused him. I am not including it to recommend this form of confrontation, nor is it provided as a sample of how such a letter "should" be written. There are many possible ways to go about confrontation — and many decisions to be made about whether direct confrontation is advisable. (For further discussion of the topic of confrontation, you may wish to look at the relevant sections in *Victims No Longer*, *The Courage to Heal*, *Half the House*, and other books). This letter is included as a reminder that old hurts don't just disappear over time, and there are ways to deal with them. It is never too late to address issues, to heal, take power, and move on with your life. What is important is not the manner of confrontation, but your commitment to moving forward regardless of the response.

Pete, 49, New York, sent me a copy of his letter along with a note that says, in part,

> "At the same time I am mailing you this note, I am mailing the attached letter. It's to my most significant childhood abuser.... A lot has changed for me in the last nine months. I wrote the attached letter. I did it!!"

I wrote back, asking Pete how he felt about my including his confrontation letter in this book, with the understanding that "it would be edited to conceal the identities of all the people and institutions you named — the good guys as well as the bad guys...." With characteristic survivor generosity (one more example of how helping others empowers the helper), Pete responded,

> "The kinds of emotions evoked by your letter are all that I've worked so hard to feel. They still feel strange but they feel SO GOOD! I would be honored that anything of mine would be even considered for use in any form of abuse recovery. Please feel free to use the letter as part of any publication, counseling, training, or other activity that might help any abuse survivor take the next step."

Later, along with his signed release form, he added,

> "I truly hope that you will decide to use my letter. Any help it could give to others would be wonderful. Makes me feel warm and strong just to think about it. Thank you."

How generous! It is Pete who deserves thanks. Here is his letter:

_____ [Last Name of Perpetrator]

My name is _____.

I recently wrote your name on a list, compiled by myself and other men. I could not remember your first name at the time for I never used it when I knew you. I do not need to use it now, even though I have looked it up.

I wrote your name on a list, identifying you as a person who had sexually abused me as a child. It was in 19__ at _____. I was fourteen years old. You were a senior, an officer, responsible for the cadets living in the dormitory above the school laundry.

I was the immature, passive, and frightened kid who still occasionally pissed in his bed. The boy who lived in the room halfway down the hall on the west side. It was the only room with a connecting opening to the next room. The adjoining room was occupied by a kid named _____. He witnessed your assaults on me and my humiliation at your hands. Do you remember?

You came at me in the dark, after lights out. Did that somehow make it OK? You tried to get me to masturbate you and I wouldn't do it. At first, you tried to cajole me. Then you threatened me with your rank and position, the authority the school had bestowed on you. The authority which made you responsible for those younger and less capable than yourself. You abused that authority and trust in the worst possible way.

When your threats didn't work, you attacked me physically. You climbed onto my bed and tried to get me to touch your penis with my hand. Each time this happened, I was able to turn over onto my stomach securing my hands and arms under me, out of your way. You became angry and, while straddling my back, you would pull one of my arms out from under me. You used your superior strength to rub my clenched fist on your erect penis, which you had exposed from your pajamas. You pried my fingers open, trying to get me to hold your penis. You insisted I masturbate you and, when I wouldn't, you would twist my arm and push it up toward my head, causing me great pain. You kept insisting that I touch your penis. You said you would stop hurting me if I did. I kept resisting and pulling away as much as possible. You kept threatening me and physically trying to get me to play with your penis. You treated me with contempt and scorn, but still you wanted and expected me to masturbate you. That was all you could think of; get your power and sexual pleasure. There was no consideration of me or my feelings, my fears, my pain, my humiliation and shame. You even had the arrogance and the shamelessness to do all that you did to me with _____ right there as a witness. You felt so superior in your actions that you did not even consider that what you were doing was wrong. You were violating ethical, cultural, and moral codes of conduct and law! You did it in front of a witness, and you did it more than once. You did it four or five times. I never gave in, but lived in terror of your next attack. My soul cried out to be left alone. All I ever wanted to do at that school was to survive.

I did. I did survive it, in spite of you and in spite of others. For a long time, I blanked out a lot of what happened to me at _____. Now I have been able to bring it all into the light of day. As part of that, I realized why you had targeted me and why you felt you could abuse me with such impunity; where your contempt and scorn had come from. I now remember seeing you with a cadet named _____ just prior to the onset of your abuse. He had sexually abused me before you. I'm sure he relayed to you his version of his abuse. He gave you the idea that you could abuse me also and not have to deal with the consequences of your actions. Well, this letter is letting you know that this is not the case.

I have been carrying guilt and shame for the abuse and humiliation at your hands for twenty-eight years. I didn't realize for many years that what you and others did to me had a very strong, negative effect on how I lived my life. It took some time and a lot of work, but I have learned that I can rid myself of that negative influence. I no longer take responsibility, nor have shame and guilt for the abuse I suffered. You especially, and others, took advantage of the artificial power structure, positions of responsibility, age, and strength to cause me physical, psychological, and sexual harm. I didn't do it. You did. I was just a young, scared kid. I didn't ask for it. I was not asked if I wanted it. I was not asked if I minded. I was not listened to when I tried to stop it. You alone are responsible, whether you accept that responsibility or not. I no longer own any of it.

As I was preparing to write this letter for the first time, I looked up your address in the school alumni directory. I never really understood until that moment why I even had one. I must have known that at some point I would want to have access to those, like yourself, who had caused me harm. When I finally looked up your name, I was shocked and horrified to discover that you were listed as a vice president of a child care and learning center. I immediately called there to see if it was true, but you had not been associated with the organization for some years. If you had been, I would have sent a copy of this letter to them also. At this point, it is enough for you to know that I no longer hold what you did to me as a secret nor as something of which I am ashamed. I have written and spoken your name to family, friends, professionals, and to other men who were also sexually abused as children. I intend to write to _____[the school], to _____[name], to inform the school through him what happened to me while I was a cadet. I do not know yet if I will name my abusers.

I do not know how you have received this letter. I do not know whether you will even read far enough to reach this point. You may deny that you know of me or what I have confronted you with. You may choose to ignore or rationalize away any involvement, or you may acknowledge your responsibility, in a healthy or in an unhealthy way. That is up to you. I have no control over that and do not want any. Regardless of how you react, I have no interest in hearing a response from you. I am moving ahead with my life and you can no longer cause me any harm, either by what has happened in the past or by any action you might choose to take in reaction to this letter. I have nothing to hide or to hide from. Friends, family, and caring professionals have supported and encouraged me in the writing of this letter. You can no longer do me any harm. You only have to live with yourself. Anyone can find help and peace if they are willing to work for it.

I have not included a return address. I have no desire to have any contact with you now or in the future. You did not respect my needs or desires twenty-eight years ago. You have this small opportunity to do so now.

Alive, strong and free,

_____[Pete's Signature]

Pete said, "I did it!" I think most people who read his words would agree.

LIMITS AND BOUNDARIES

In addition to confrontation (sometimes as part of it) attention is being paid to the importance of reasonable limits. Respecting his own pace, intensity, and limits is evidence of the survivor's growing self-awareness. He is able to stand up for what he needs. References are made to setting *safe boundaries*, including *sexual boundaries.*

> "...decent touch...whenever a hint of the grasping hands looms, tears flow freely as I practice recalling the banishing." — Lawrence, 62, New York

> "...respecting my own boundaries. I am learning that I am valuable and that my boundaries *deserve* respect. When I respect my own boundaries, the natural result is respect for others' boundaries as well." — Geoffrey, 32 Colorado

> "I can say no to sex. I can say yes. I have a choice." — Val, 30, Florida

◆ ◆ ◆ ◆ ◆

This lovely, powerful poem was written by **Rob, 38, Ohio**. One summer evening, he read it to twenty-nine other men gathered on a wooded ridge top. We watched Rob appear to grow stronger and more confident as his proclamation touched twenty-nine hearts:

Be gone from my bed, you foes that don't belong there
I choose rather to find comfort
in peace, beauty, serenity,
and true love.
I have the power now to
fill my mind with gentler thoughts
and my heart with a warmth
of purer and more genuine connections I am making

Be gone from my bed, you foes that don't belong there
I never invited you in, or if I did
it was without knowing the liar, the trickster that you were
I am on to you now

Be gone from my bed, you foes that don't belong there
This is now a safe place
reserved only for peace
and beautiful acts of love.

Be gone from my bed, you foes that don't belong there
I have allies now
They have taught me well
You do not have the power I once gave you

Be gone from my bed, you foes that don't belong there
You know you don't belong there
and you know who you are
You know you don't belong here

I have cried so many times, tears on the inside
from stories I thought I never could tell.
The words are flowing now.
And so comes the tears.
My pain is leaving
and so are my fears
and I am singing
I am not alone
I AM NOT ALONE.

Be gone from my bed, you foes that don't belong there
I used to high drink work buzz sex think you away

That was a game
but now this part is real

Be gone from my bed, you foes that don't belong there
I have pride; it keeps you away
I have respect; it keeps you away
I have friendship; it keeps you away
I am loved; I forgive you some
but you're still not welcome in my bed
or my safe places

Be gone from my bed, you foes that don't belong there

BE GONE

As part of their new understanding of limits and boundaries, some men stress the importance of *listening* — to themselves and to others.

> "...taking care of myself and listening to other survivors..." — Bob, 57, North Dakota

> "...developing myself as an active listener — I trained and am active in...a crisis telephone line." — Bob, 65, Delaware

Others write of their need to *maintain distance* from some or all family members.

> "...staying away from family of origin." — Jon, 53, Kentucky

> "I have had to cease contact with my family of origin.... [They] continue in their denial and dysfunction.... I cannot have my life on hold waiting.... Recovery has taught me that I deserve love and that I am capable of returning it. Today, my wife is a part of that cycle, as are my friends, male and female, as am I. While I still love my family, [theirs] is a cycle broken by pain and mired in fear." — John, 32, Newfoundland, Canada

ATTENTION TO SELF

This is the area where I notice the most powerful growth. Many of the statements indicate tremendous increase in *self-respect, self-care,* and, above all, *self-confidence.*

> "...myself and on the fact that I am getting this behind me and that I am not letting this control my life." — David, 35, Wyoming

> "...respect of myself and all that I have accomplished..." — Carlos, 47, Peru

> "...myself. My previous support systems weren't enough for me anymore.... I needed to rely on Me in order to progress in my health and recovery...it was a big risk to rely on me for my support, even though it seems like the natural place to find it." — Bob, 45, New York

> "...taking care of myself..." — Xandu the Giant, 33, New York

> "...my needs. Taking care of Mark because I do count...I am a worthwhile and good person." — Mark, 34, West Virginia

> "...myself, my accomplishments (of which I now see there are many), my good points (as opposed to just the bad), and the positive directions I am taking myself, as well as those I would like to investigate in the future." — Michael, 31, New York

> "...my confidence that I can see it through, wherever the path takes me. I have the strength, understanding, and support. No turning back. My direction is forward." — Les, 60, New Zealand

Responses show a profound *commitment* to self, and to continuing to make *healthy life changes.*

> "...looking after 'me' for a change. By becoming more self-accepting, I have been able to *slowly* lose the sense of responsibility I feel." — Barry, 38 Ontario, Canada

"...making time for myself." — Jerry, 47, Nova Scotia, Canada

"...myself. I've given up trying to get the perpetrators to take responsibility. As Mike said at the survivors' workshop, 'As long as recovery depends on someone else's response, they have the power.' " — Kevin, 35, Pennsylvania

By late recovery, self-focus no longer is about survival; it concerns *growth* and *change*.

"...strengthening my gay identity..." — Mike, 51, Ohio

"I keep on surprising myself at how far I have come." — Jim, 58, Kansas

"...to be able to change, grow, and learn." — Xandu the Giant, 33, New York

"...taking full control of and responsibility for my life; in particular, safely exploring my sexuality, writing poetry and literature, composing music, painting (art), safe contact with supportive and trustworthy friends, and activism (writing letters, giving interviews, calling talk shows) in favor of incest survivors and the issues we face in recovery and coping with life." — Rick, 47, Massachusetts

The *subtleties* and shadings of life are being noticed and appreciated.

"...recognizing my normalcy...I have been very active in pulling myself back from the pit before it gets really bad." — Dan, 34, Ontario, Canada

"...to love me...to see things not only in black and white." — Michael, 46, North Carolina

Past hurts have been put into *perspective*.

"...daily check-in on how far I've come, and that I'm not immune to other problems or relapse into old survival defenses." — Pete, 49, New York

"...remembering how far I've come, and the freedom created by getting better." — Rick, 35, North Carolina

Enormous healing has taken place.

> **"I keep my focus on the fact that I am a special person and that my experience as a survivor of sexual child abuse can take a positive dimension. I can go on with my life. All my work in therapy has allowed me to grieve my past. Life can be beautiful and I can let my inner child play." — Daniel, 39, New Brunswick and Ontario, Canada**

Life has become more complete and desirable.

> **"...living my life to the fullest." — Patrick, 42, Rhode Island**

> **"...Free Choice. I choose to live a healthy life. My life is filled with riches." — Magnus, 37, Sweden**

Responses in this area (attention to self) have moved beyond trying to summon sufficient inner strength to endure the fears of daily living and the terrors of the night. That part is over; those wounds have healed.

> **"...opening up, sharing myself with others." — Bill, 52, Massachusetts**

Survivors now concentrate on self-*exploration*, self-*appreciation*, self-*affirmation*, and self-*development*.

> **"...understanding myself more. What triggers my feelings? What underlying beliefs have I developed that motivate my thoughts, feelings, actions? Who am I?" — Rick, 35, Montana**

> **"...living each day for myself and knowing that I am a stronger, better person today." — Dan, 28, Massachusetts**

> **"...trying to discover the real beautiful me." — Rich, 30, New York**

> **"...I deserve love and self-respect." — Steven, 37, New York**

> **"...the better me I can create..." — Fred, 20, New Jersey**

Dozens of responses take this direction. Even more strongly than self-*appreciation*, male survivors write of self-*love* and self-*nurturing*.

> **"...loving myself." — Stan, 47, Indiana**

> "...openly acknowledging that I am a survivor of incest, to stay with that truth, and to love myself through having my feelings and to be able to live with that truth." — Peter, 37, Massachusetts

> "...loving myself and doing what makes me happy." — Angelo, 25, Massachusetts

> "...taking better overall care of myself in all aspects. Incest is not often a focus anymore, thankfully. Back then I never thought I'd ever say that. I assist my recovery today by loving myself at all times. I can do that now. There is no part of me that I neglect anymore." — Jim, 35, Maine

They acknowledge their newly discovered (and newly trusted) ability to set and maintain reasonable, healthy *boundaries*, respect their own *paces*, and be *gentle* with themselves.

> "...having found my limits and not feeling I have to rush beyond them." — Bill, 40, County Strathclyde, Scotland

> "...moving at my own pace..." — Stephen, 34, California

> "...being kind to myself." — John, 43, Maryland

> "...being gentle with myself and my recovery. I let it evolve as I am ready and willing. When emotions and flashbacks come up, writing my feelings helps get them out. When there are people I can ask for help, it is opening up to ask for support." — Bill, 38, Alaska

These responses are a continuing reminder that, for many of us, there is no greater challenge than *letting ourselves off the hook*, and no greater triumph than when it is achieved. Once this feat has been accomplished, the whole world looks and feels quite different.

> "...to some extent...I don't think you ever stop healing, but the intensity of the process seems to lessen with time — so I always remind myself that the process continues and will continue. By acknowledging this I allow myself to feel human. I can make a mistake without beating myself up." — Mark, 34, Alberta, Canada

> "Mostly, I live in accord with my gifts, desires, and spiritual source. Creating and celebrating life." —Treetop, 40, Arizona

> "...the new man who is just starting his journey..." — John, 38, Oklahoma

> "I focus on me, a man, a gay man who has things to contribute to life. Life is a buffet; if you sit on the sidelines, you're going to starve. I used to be this person who would sit and watch folks go by. Now I go out and TALK to folks.... I spent the first twenty-five years in hell; the next twenty-five are MINE, not theirs. I also have to remind myself that I am good at surviving. LIVING, however, is a new skill that I am learning — and learning to enjoy. I feel like this is a new me slowly emerging from a cocoon. Don't know what will turn out, but the process is interesting." — Benn, 32, Pennsylvania

This important undertaking — learning to be easier on himself — extends to the survivor's appreciative recognition of the bravery, innocence, and goodness of *the child he was.* Response after response reveals dedication to loving, protecting, and nurturing that "*inner child.*"

> "...listening to the little boy who knew, and loving and caring for him." — Ken, 44, Ontario, Canada

> "...the poor little boys who live on in me, and adhere to the promise I made them that, despite the agony, I would go back in time to rescue them and make them whole." — Paddy, 49, Queensland, Australia

> "I am certain in myself that working on my wounded inner child offers me the most positive way forward." — Don [no age given], Yorkshire, England

> "...taking care of my Inner Child." — Joe, 56, Florida

I have heard people express annoyance with the concept of "inner child work," seeing it as regressive or infantile. There are those who reject it as resistance to growing up — avoiding responsibility for one's life. Some take the concept literally, and others understand it as a metaphor. I understand the "Inner Child" to be that amazing spark that clings to the essence of humanity in the face of discouragement and hurt. Inner child work helps survivors understand the reality of who they were, what happened to them, and how they survived. Loving the child you were is a major step toward loving the person you became.

Several survivors with histories of *dissociation* or multiplicity/dissociative identity extend their self-affirmation to *creating safety* for their dissociation, *accepting, encouraging,* and eventually *integrating their alters.*

> "...trying to keep myself safe emotionally, so that my inner persons can feel safe enough to reveal themselves...I found a medium for my alters to begin expressing themselves...movement and dance." — Zandy, 44, New Jersey

> "...staying in contact with the 'hurt children' inside of me and providing them nurturing and support..." — Jim, 55, Michigan

> "...cooperation — I'm a multiple." — Iceman, 20, Illinois

> "...integration of my alters, recognition and reparenting of my inner child, integration with daily living and the constant fight of keeping back denial. — Larry, 32, New York

In every way (and in ever-increasing numbers) these men in late stages of recovery write of *commitment* to themselves and to life. They take *responsibility* for their own lives and for their *behavior.*

> "...being responsible for my own healing, happiness, and well-being. Even though I've held them all accountable, I nonetheless must get on with my life." — Michael, 30, Ohio

> "...learning as much about life as I can. I understand that my feelings are important and that my children depend on me for a father figure to learn from." — Christopher, 33, Victoria, Australia

> "...taking ownership for my own activities, and recognizing that as bad as the abuse still feels, it was not and is not all of my life, all that happened to me..." — Oliver, 53, Massachusetts

They write about creating successful *change*, changing their *behavior*, *habits*, *reactions*, and *beliefs*. *Change* — exciting, important and lasting.

> "...changing those things that I do have control over." — Steven, 26, New Hampshire

> "...[I] have quit smoking, stopped all antidepressants, and recently knocked off the caffeine and minor tranquilizers. Not easy or comfortable, but the payoff is beginning to be a much clearer and more focused mind. Still shaky. I've done this only under supervision of a psychiatrist." — Timothy, 37, Alabama

> "...changing reactions and fears that are no longer appropriate, e.g., this is *not* my mother, and this is *not* my fault." — Dave, 52, Massachusetts

> "...changing my belief that the abuse was my fault!" — Sam, 26, Virginia

> "...staying in touch...being as honest as I can with others about how I feel. That includes liking myself (which helps me like and trust others) and 'lightening up.' I play when I can, and find that others don't run away when I do. Often they play with me." — John, 58, Washington, D.C.

Following a weekend male survivors' workshop, **Rob, 38, Ohio,** sent a letter to the other participants. It read, in part:

> **Dear Gentle Men,**
>
> **I am writing to inform you that I have changed I am Treating myself better, and a bit less anguished Thank you....**
> **I try to remember to notice the colors And how strong and powerful a gang you are. Thank you.**
>
> **When I got home to _____ I burned the lists of perps [names of perpetrators] On my charcoal grill**
>
> **It smelled awful**

But it felt great

I hope we meet again soon

With love, hope, and fondness,

Rob

◆ ◆ ◆ ◆ ◆

An excerpt from the poem, **"Mom Died"** by **John, 38, Alaska,** provides an appropriate ending to this section:

> **A voice within me says**
> **   extend a helping hand.**
> **   transcend self to assist others help themselves.**
> **   open my unconditional love.**
> **   realize to love oneself is unconditional love.**
> **   be gentle with myself first.**

Where originates this voice?
**   Can I really listen to it?**
**   Will I trust its advice?**

The power of unconditional love is beyond my comprehension,
*   though I felt it stirring*
*   as I held her hand.*

> *Now I focus on reforging my body,*
>
> *   my mind,*
>
> *   my spirit.*

◆ ◆ ◆ ◆ ◆

ATTENTION TO OTHERS

Along with the striking increase in paying positive attention to self, there is a huge flowering of *concern for others*.

"...giving hope to others..." — Brent, 35, Oklahoma

In some instances, concern is manifested by greater interest in the needs of the *people in the survivor's immediate life*.

> "...being sensitive to others — my partner, my children, the people I work with." — George, 43, Nova Scotia, Canada

Others move further afield.

> "I help others, both professionally and otherwise, in their effort to seek relief from the consequences of sexual abuse." — Roger, 44, Florida

> "...looking for a way to help others discover themselves." — David, 61, Michigan

For some men, it takes the form of *giving back*, repaying the help they received during the difficult years of survival and recovery. It may involve *good works* specifically for victims, or more general helping activities.

> "...learning all I can about this last great taboo and developing the skills required to help other victims." — Paul, 43, County Devon, England

> "I am training as a teacher in...dance therapy — tailor-made for survivors." — Billy, 42, County Avon, England

> "...to reach out to my brother and sister survivors and offer them some of what was given to me." — Ray, 34, Idaho

At times there is *advocacy* in the area of *child protection, general* or *personal* (in the form of good parenting), creation of *services for survivors*, or working to *humanize laws* concerning sexual child abuse.

> "...living openly, being truthful, reaching out to help kids in distress." — Robert, 46, California

> "...bringing up my daughter. Bringing up a child who is valued, respected, loved, and encouraged to grow into a responsible, caring adult is my way of getting revenge against all the people who degraded me and abused me." — Jon, 47, Minnesota

> "...trying to slow down and be more *here* with my children." — Ira, 44, New York

> "...developing resources for both men and women and through the help that I offer to other survivors and friends

I learn to better understand and accept myself and change a victimization into strengthening experience and thus conquering the abuse." — Pierre, 28, New Brunswick/Nouveau-Brunswick, Canada

◆ ◆ ◆ ◆ ◆

One example of survivors *making a difference within their own communities* follows. **Jerry, 47, Nova Scotia, Canada,** sent a response that included a flyer and letter that read, in part,

"Two other male survivors and myself have started a support group. The group is called S.A.M.S. (Sexually Abused Males Surviving). We have been going for over a year now, and things are going quite well."

The flyer for the group is simple and to the point. It is brightly colored and bears the image of an eagle flying. Here is the text:

S.A.M.S.
Sexually Abused Males Surviving

SAMS is a self-help support group for men who have suffered childhood sexual abuse, or any other type of sexual abuse.

FOUNDED BY SURVIVORS FOR SURVIVORS

New members are welcomed to a safe and comfortable place where they can gain support, understanding, acceptance, and knowledge regarding sexual abuse. Following is a brief outline of the purpose and mission of SAMS.

"OUR PURPOSE" To help all male victims of sexual abuse learn how to deal effectively with the aftermath of the abuse and thereby become the truly whole person they were meant to be in the beginning.

"OUR MISSION" To meet on a regular basis at a regular time providing a safe and comfortable place for men to share and support one another in *complete confidentiality*. To provide an organization dedicated to researching and maintaining information to assist surviving men. To help all members truly apply the term *self-help* and achieve their maximum level of personal growth and development.

Being a victim of childhood sexual abuse can lead to a myriad of problems such as substance abuse, sexual identity problems, phobias, panic disorders, depression, relationship dysfunctions, etc., etc. (and many many more).

THESE PROBLEMS CANNOT AND SHOULD NOT BE DEALT WITH ALONE. WE CAN HELP!

Currently the best estimate is that one in six boys are sexually abused prior to age fourteen.

Those that understand have the best chance of instituting change.

If you feel this group may be for you, please join now.

"To those who succumbed to the pain, we will never forget your silent screams. To those who struggle to thrive in our midst, embrace your secrets and BE SILENT NO LONGER."
— by Fred Tolson, author and founder of M.A.L.E.

The remainder of the flyer lets people know how to obtain more information. Nothing elaborate — the whole thing fits on a single sheet of paper. But it doesn't take more than that to make a difference. If you want to create change in your community, think of what you want to say and do. Then do it in your own way. Jerry and his friends did.

Whether in the form of aiding victims, working with other survivors or engaging in other helping activities during late recovery, male survivors find new energy and commitment to speaking out.

Another example of grass roots activism by male survivors came from **Chris, 45, Florida**. He and his organization, The Alpha Foundation ("...committed to the protection of boys who are abused and healing the men they become"), work to increase public awareness of male survivor issues. In his letter, Chris wrote, "Recently, I requested an executive order be issued by the Mayor of West Palm Beach...declaring the second Saturday of each April as MALE SEXUAL ABUSE AWARENESS DAY.... Mayor Graham...was supportive.... Instead of limiting the scope of the proclamation to a single day...she surprised us by making the proclamation cover the entire month of April.... As of this writing, a second proclamation was issued by the mayor of Largo, Florida.... It was easy to get the proclamation from our Mayor — all we did was mail her a request letter...you, and the male survivors in your area (can) do the same." (For further information, contact The Alpha Foundation — see the Resource Section.) The text of the Mayor's Proclamation follows:

◆ ◆ ◆ ◆ ◆

The City of West Palm Beach
PROCLAMATION

WHEREAS, whether by simple neglect or conspiracy, the problem of child sexual abuse persists in an atmosphere of silence and ignorance; and

WHEREAS, any community, organization, or individual who attempts to remain neutral or fails to support the protection of all children from sexual exploitation is at least passively supportive of continued sexual exploitation; and

WHEREAS, as compared with female children who are victimized, the problem of boyhood sexual exploitation is more often overlooked, neglected, and poorly understood; and

WHEREAS, while efforts to protect girls from sexual victimization and rehabilitative services provided to those who are traumatized are well underway, collectively applying these same efforts on behalf of male children has lagged; and

WHEREAS, boys who are sexually abused usually lack appropriate male role models and mentors to assist them in their recovery, provide support during any prosecution, and advocate on their behalf with other adults and organizations and as a result sustain additional trauma and suffer developmentally; and

WHEREAS, it is encouraged that all adult survivors, especially male, provide appropriate nurturing, support, and guidance to sexual abuse victims as they are able; and

WHEREAS, all adult survivors, advocate for the prevention of childhood sexual abuse and for the development of effective and comprehensive recovery and rehabilitative programs for victims within the limits of his or her governmental and cultural restrictions and to the extent he or she is able.

NOW THEREFORE, I, Nancy M. Graham, Mayor of the City of West Palm Beach, Florida, do hereby proclaim the month of April 1998 as:

MALE SEXUAL ABUSE AWARENESS MONTH

in the City of West Palm Beach, Florida.

IN WITNESS WHEREOF, I hereunto set my hand and cause the official seal of the City of West Palm Beach, Florida to be affixed this 23rd day of February, 1998.

(Signed) Nancy M. Graham
Mayor

More and more, through education, advocacy, political, or social action, male survivors are using their recovered strength to help change the world.

> "...the process of breathing new life into my soul is a committed ongoing process. I speak out freely today of male sexual abuse whenever God gives me the opportunity." — Brent, 48, Utah

> "...taking action..." — Aaron, 29, New Mexico

> "...revealing my gifts." — Davis, 54, Ohio

> "I had felt without power. Today I believe you, Mike, when you say that we are creating a new world." — Jose, 41, Argentina

RELIGION AND SPIRITUALITY

Widening interest in the world beyond the individual (and beyond the hurt) may extend to *spiritual* or *religious exploration*.

> "...knowing the wonder of all Creation...the Holy Spirit in every living thing." — Luis, 35, Colombia

> "...my spiritual path — unconditional love." — Nick, 47, Texas

Trusting his sense of rightness, the male survivor has gained greater freedom to explore what *healthy spirituality* means to him. The increase isn't dramatic, but from mid-stage to late recovery there are more responses concerning *religion* and *spirituality*.

> "...my spiritual life — to free me of other problems after the crisis stage." — Bill, 50, Vermont

> "...myself and the God of my understanding." — Brad, 43, Florida

> "...increasingly, spiritual experience..." — Douglas, 45, Czech Republic

Few men speak of organized religion and none mentions members of the clergy. But there is renewed emphasis on *faith, religion, religious teachings*, and *spirituality*.

> "...*my* faith. It isn't the religion I was raised up in, but I feel I am closer to truly understanding what religion is about." — Randy, 36, Tennessee

> "...finding peace through the Scriptures." — Brent, 35, Oklahoma

> "...the bedrock which has always been my source of strength over the past seven years, a spiritual faith. It fits no clear denomination or tradition (Christian, Zen, Monastic, Buddhism, etc.), but it feeds me in a way nothing else does. Now have begun daily meditations in the morning...took a long time and a lot of work to get to the point of being able to relax without panic attacks. VERY NICE SPACE. Goal is now to begin to carve out time at the end of the day for some silence and stillness." — Timothy, 37, Alabama

References to *Higher Power, God,* or "*God Within*" remain constant.

> "I could tap into a source of strength and unclouded support that wouldn't wear out, move away, get frustrated or

angry, and wasn't damaged from past abuse. Therefore...a relationship with God through His teachings in the Bible..." — Doug, 35, California

"...the God within me." — Eston, 43, Kentucky

Along with fewer references to *prayer* and *devotions*, we see greater interest in *meditation*.

"...prayer...is my greatest source of vision and energy to do truly new and big things I would never have done before..." — Bill, 45, Delaware

"...meditation which anchors me in the moment, emphasizes impermanence, and teaches compassion." — Doug, 46, New York

"...meditation, my spiritual practice, is the strongest support I have." — David, 57, New Mexico

Here is the poem by **Keith, 31, Quebec, Canada,** that I promised you earlier. Keith provides us with a wonderful metaphor of the power of recovery in the company of other survivors, his faith and the successful result of his risk-taking. For readers who are unfamiliar with the reference, *Maid of the Mist* is a boat that takes visitors to view the base of Niagara Falls.

Maid of the Mist

And sixty-five of us, all dressed alike,
Gather on the deck of this tiny boat,
Pondering the insanity that brought us here.
Green water churns and boils beneath us, all around:
Whirlpools, raging rapids, and undertow.
We do not move...we bob, we toss, we roll,
But do not move.
Two diesel engines roar, full power,
It's all they can do to fight the flow.
And water tumbles down from thirty times our height
A drop, a cup, a billion barrels a second,
Raising a spray that rolls in droplets down our cheeks

And falls from our chins into the torrent below.
People look down from the rim of the gorge
(How far away they appear)
And see rainbows over our boat
And say how it looks like a rough ride.
But they, who have never been in it,
How could they ever know
That we must cling to one another
Just to keep from falling into the Maelstrom.
We look around and see only spray,
And falling water, and falling water,
And falling water and sheer rock cliff,
And the cabin of our boat...
The wheelhouse...the Captain...
We must put our lives in the hands
Of the Captain
His hands, steady on the wheel,
Will guide us safely through,
For He has piloted these waters before.
He knows the rocks, the currents, the eddies,
And the Safe Passage.
He has brought many through before,
And many shall come through with Him again.
He is in this boat with us
And only He can be in Control.
Oh, God, how hard it is to let go and
Trust the Captain.
In His hands, we shall soon stand
On firm, dry, unmoving ground,
And look back upon our experiences here:
Compare our perceptions, thoughts, and feelings
And only have to say: "WOW!"

◆ ◆ ◆ ◆ ◆

INTERPERSONAL EXPLORATION

Renewed confidence, an outgrowth of successful recovery, is
expressed through exploration. Responses include *exploring sexuality*

and *sexual identity, intimacy, dating, relationships,* and *risk-taking* in general.

> "...the intimacy issues raised by being in a relationship with my boyfriend. The relationship is teaching me that sex is not the demeaning, degrading, and objectifying act that I learned from the sexual abuse, but rather a beautiful expression of love between two people." — Sean, 29, Massachusetts

> "I have begun to build bridges to my wife. We would never have started the process to intimacy if I had not learned the words." — Ed, 46, Minnesota

> "...[my wife] and I are talking more and reading about intimacy." — David, 54, Colorado

> "...attempting intimacy: Learning how to love in *healthy ways* that I didn't learn from my family. Taking risks...dating. 'Looking for a soul mate.'" — Xandu the Giant, 33, New York

> "...recovery in maintaining fluid boundaries and the belief in my gifts. Through these actions I maintain my power in my intimate relationship." — Jay, 40, Texas

> "...all new experiences, but I am finding myself more open to risks/uncertainties. It's exciting and scary at the same time. — Frank, 28, Virginia

◆ ◆ ◆ ◆ ◆

John, 38, Alaska, offered a number of his moving poems for inclusion in this book. I chose "Intimacy, Part Two," a stirring presentation of how, years after suffering abuse by his mother, he repaired his ability to trust while exploring boundaries.

Intimacy
Part Two

Her fingers glide gingerly along my arm,
  My fingers glide gingerly along her arm.
    Her fingers tenderly touch my chest,
      My fingers tenderly touch her chest.

Her fingers tickle my toes,
My fingers tickle her toes.

Together we explore.
Together we share.
Together we trust.
We trust the other.
We trust ourselves.
We trust our union.

Her fingers walk across my stomach,
I ask her to stop short.
To stop short of my boundary,
My boundary for intimacy at this moment.
My moment of wanting the rest of me for me,
Our shared and respected boundary.

She agrees.   Her fingers stop short.

My fingers ask,
Ask about mutual respect,
Ask about mutual trust,
Ask about her boundaries.

With tenderness she helps me understand.
Understand that not all women violate men,
As my mother violated me.

With tenderness she helps me relearn trust,
With tenderness she helps me relearn respect,
With tenderness I help me relearn love.

With tenderness we relearn the pleasure of pleasure.
Pleasure of trusting the fingers will stop short.
Pleasure of respecting each other's wishes.
Pleasure of trusting touch.
Pleasure of shared peacefulness.
Pleasure of caring.

Caring for my body,
Caring for me,

Caring.
So simple.
So difficult.
So essential.

We create gentle feelings,
We create gentleness full of caring,
A caring so strong,
Strong as a baby's grip,
Strong as a baby's breath,
Strong as a baby's love.

With her help
With her patience
With her gentleness
With her openness
With her caring—With my trust,
We come together.

With my willingness,
With my fears,
With my hope,
With my faith,

We come together in a sensual way.
We come together in a convincing way,
We come together in healing way,
We come together in trusting way,
We come together in a way that convinces me
sex is superfluous.

We come together with intimacy,
Intimacy.
Shared trust.
Shared caring.
Shared love.

Intimacy.
In-to-me-you-see.
In-to-her-you-see.
In-to-us-you-see.

Intimacy,
The ultimate intercourse,
The ultimate sensual experience.

◆ ◆ ◆ ◆ ◆

FORGIVENESS

Forgiveness is a difficult and tricky concept, having many different meanings. This may be why it doesn't make sense to address the subject during early stages of recovery — too much risk of falling prey to confusion, denial, pretense, wishful thinking, or other people's agendas. There is a great deal of work to be done before a survivor is free to deal with what forgiveness means to him. Further along, in late recovery, a few survivors begin to bring up the subject in its many forms, including "*heartfelt forgiveness*," *self-forgiveness*, and *non-forgiveness.*

> "...the letter from my perpetrator asking for forgiveness of the awful SIN. And me in my heart forgiving them." — Mark, 30, Louisiana

> "...continuing to forgive myself." — John, 38, Oklahoma

> "...forgiving myself and embracing the little kid in me and protecting him." — Red, 39, Ontario, Canada

> "...knowing that I don't have to forgive! I also don't have to carry the pain and a grudge any longer. Today I concentrate on letting go of my anger, and thus no longer empower the incest of my youth. What happened will always be there, but I no longer have to let it dominate my life. I have found the power, that was always within me, to move beyond incest." — Chris, 57, Ohio

THE ROLE OF FEELINGS

The level of acceptance of *feelings* has risen dramatically.

> "...my feelings." — Randy, 35, California

> "Recently in therapy I have been able to feel and sob about the deep sadness by playing 'Go Fish,' a children's game.... My energy level seemed to be higher after this occurred. I danced with my sixteen-month-old daughter to the music on the radio." — Mark, 30, Indiana

No longer threatened by their emotions, having worked through years of fear and anger, in late recovery, male survivors incorporate expression of feelings as part of a healthy, integrated life.

> "...trying to focus less on *thinking* about what happened and more on *feeling*, both the past and the present." — Bob, 43, California

> "...allowing myself to feel." — Bob, 46, Ontario, Canada

With this acceptance comes understanding that the purpose of feelings is to be felt, not feared or avoided.

> "...learning to verbalize what I'm feeling and sometimes just sitting in those feelings until they pass, and they *do* pass." — Aaron, 29, New Mexico

> "...what is important in my life...I have the courage to tell how I'm feeling, and to act on my needs. I have begun to recognize my anger as a residual feeling from my abuse, and am beginning to learn how to hold the anger for an appropriate moment. I am beginning to feel how my parents must have felt, as they covered up their feelings in a decorative package for the world to see, and then lost all conscious connection with their insides." — Ed, 46, Minnesota

> "...stopping to ask myself what I'm feeling, taking those feelings seriously, and having compassion for them." — Tim, 32, Connecticut

Thus, there is a huge increase in general references to *expressing feelings*, along with greater acceptance of *crying* or *grieving* (including recovering the ability to cry), or simply regaining the *ability to feel*.

> "...letting *all* my feelings out! — Will, 55, Arkansas

> "...grief work...work with anger." — Mike, 51, Ohio

> "...growing through grief and change..." — Ram, 50, Manitoba, Canada

> "...after the tears comes laughter." — Hector, 58, Mexico

> "...getting in touch with feelings that were there in me, somewhere among that pain and numbing. These were

> not able to develop [when] I was a child." — Ron, 52, Missouri

In addition, we find new references to expressing *anger* as well as *laughter* and *joy*.

> "...self-respect, and the rightness of my anger." — Mike, 37, Prince Edward Island, Canada

> "...anger work! And shame and a lot of other emotions, through therapy." — Pete, 30, California

> "...my sense of humor. My laughter allows me to cry and my tears allow me to laugh. Love of paradox?" — William, 46, Arizona

> "...sometimes we laugh till our sides hurt." — Tom, 61, Maine

◆ ◆ ◆ ◆ ◆

Relaxing and reclaiming their sense of humor show up everywhere. Here is another example of how it is possible — and sometimes necessary — to treat heavy topics with a light touch. Five male survivors (**Bill, 40, Nebraska; Jim, 32, Maryland; Len, 50, Pennsylvania; Rick, 41, New Jersey;** and **Tom, 44, Pennsylvania**) performed this song at a weekend workshop. They rewrote the words and sang it to the tune of the old American standard, "Take Me Out to the Ball Game":

> Take me out of this mind game.
> Take me out of this game.
> Don't touch my peanuts,
> I'll crack you, Jack.
> Go away and don't ever come back.
>
> With this group and our home team
> We're gonna win, Fuck the shame.
> For it's one, two, three strikes, no outs
> And there's no mind game.

◆ ◆ ◆ ◆ ◆

People often tell me that they are surprised at the amount of laughter and humor at my workshops and professional trainings. They wonder how I can address such heavy topics so lightly. I reply that I don't know any other way to approach the depths of fear, anger, grief, and shame without shutting everyone down. There is an enormous difference between using jokes to insult, belittle, tease, or shame, and laughing at a situation to rise above feelings of despair and hopelessness. Persecuted and misunderstood people have always used humor in this way — Jews in the ghetto and during the Holocaust, African-Americans during slavery, and many other oppressed groups. Similarly, survivors and their allies are forging a humor of recovery. The times of taunting and mocking are over; humor is not being employed to hide the painful realities of abuse. Laughter is taking its rightful place in healing, alongside all the other expressions of emotion. All these feelings can be aspects of what one man called his *"shame work."* Although it is certainly possible to feel bad, there is no such thing as a "bad feeling." What is bad is numbness — the absence of feelings. When painful feelings are expressed, the pain diminishes and healing occurs; if emotions are deadened by numbness, the hurt continues. Let your feelings flow.

This poem, a celebration of feelings and the senses, was sent by **Christopher, 33, Victoria, Australia**:

A Brand-New Day

Yea, this is the way I want to feel, waking to a brand-new day.
Clear blue skies with golden rays to tingle my skin, a great way to begin.
I'm excited at nothing but just to be alive.
It's easy to find something to do when I'm not feeling blue.
I'll bake a cake and think of how it will taste.
I'll listen to songs and won't think of wrongs.
I'm pleased that I can feel this way and I'm happy to see that you're looking at me, content to just let it be.

Participants at some weekend workshops can choose to work with a large punching bag as a means of encouraging their emotional expression. Some readers no doubt remember this experience. For those who haven't tried it, this poem conveys its power perfectly. It was written by **John, 58, Washington, D.C.**:

...JUST A BAG HANGING FROM THE CEILING.

That's all it is,
        hanging by silvery chains
        from a padeye in the beam
        of an old farmhouse ceiling.

        White with red
        and blue trim
        "Everlast"
...hanging still in the air.

It was there when the men came in:
Quietly, tensely, with
expectations, and fears, and
angers.
The bag, hanging from the ceiling
...that's all it is.

With a sense of love and care for each other,
The men focused
Their angers, their fears, their disappointments,
Their rages, their tears, their abandonments
...on the bag, hanging still from the ceiling.

The first man swung
        three times—
But with what power
and accuracy he aimed.

With a roar he slammed
the ax handle in the middle
        of the bag.
His roar resonated
with all the watching men,
with a force to keep it
rolling round the room.
The bag, no longer still,
rocked and swayed before his power.

Three times he swung the bat...
Three times the bag swayed
        and rocked.

Three times his rage was roared
'round the room among the men.

And then there was silence.

In the center of the group
of silent and focused men

...just a bag was hanging,
still, from the ceiling.

What was the bag for the man?
What demons did it face for him?

An abusing mother? an absent father?
a careless neighbor?
a punishing grandmother?
a drunken uncle? a bullying brother?
a demanding sister?
a lying and selfish poser of a friend?

No matter which, or none,
or even the sum of all...
the bag was the focus,
and for the moment took
the rage, the hurt, the disappointment,
the fears, the tears, the expectations
of the first man...

All, all could be in that bag,
...hanging from the ceiling.

And the men who followed him that afternoon
were cheered on by their brothers,
inspired to swing their fears
and tears and abandonments
down the bat and into the bag
...hanging from the ceiling.

The bag swayed and rocked
and once steadied was
ready to take more.

None but the first man
and those who followed him

will know what they left behind—
and what power they carried away.

The rage that resounded
around the room,
the roars that rolled
out over the valley and up the hill,
gave power and focus to the pain...
So unfairly given, so truly felt
...in bones, in guts, in muscle.

How much the bag took...
only the men who aimed and
swung, roared and hit
will ever know
...but it rocked and swayed
in time to their blows.

The men have gone.
The bag still hangs
in the middle of the farmhouse room.

It is just a bag
...hanging from the ceiling.

TRUST

Barriers built of fear, hurt, and suspicion — walls of mistrust —
crumble. Tentatively, but courageously and inexorably, male survivors
begin to *trust* themselves and others.

> "...putting my health first. Listening to the voice inside
> me; knowing that it knows which direction I need to
> take." — Michael, County Dublin, Ireland

> "...how to identify and appropriately express my feelings.
> I have learned to trust my own intuition." — Steve, 42,
> South Dakota

> "...realizing that it really did happen and refraining from
> denying it...[I] reveal the incest to the women I go out
> with...most of the time [they] have been more compas-
> sionate after I opened myself up." — Chris, 22, Texas

Nothing will ever again be the same for these brave men.

HOPE, GRACE, AND MOVING ON

This is the second poem sent by **Eston, 43, Kentucky**:

Grace

The impression is upon me;
The resilience of love everlasting
With an aurora none can see
Yet its shadow forever casting.
For love is not lost in place nor day.
It is ever present to reveal
The most worthy possession we give away,
And inherited by those who will.
As it will be so unto death
And yet on for those who know;
Let them keep warm in the aftermath
Our hearts with affection will bestow.

◆ ◆ ◆ ◆ ◆

Hope has returned. Free from the tyranny of past injuries, these male survivors *move on* with *hope* and *confidence*.

"...taking care of myself (it's OK to say NO), nurturing my inner child, and getting on with my life — moving on from survivor to thriver." — Curt, 43, Wisconsin

"My work now is not about compensating for the past, but transcendence. I feel very grateful for all the experiences that shaped me and led me to where I am today, and to the power and possibilities it opened up to me. It was worth it. I'd choose it all over again. The process of recovery requires that we open ourselves to our feelings, and learn to listen to what our bodies tell us. It makes us wise and strong, people of power and joy. So, I guess that's what I focus on — what do I feel right now." — Olin, 42, Vermont

For the first time, the men write about *relaxation*, *enjoyment*, moving positively and confidently into the *future*.

"I try to take life easy. For the moment I've cooled down the incest part." — Hamid, 52, Denmark

"...my needs and enjoying my life..." — Paul, 41, New York

"...all the positive changes I am seeing as I go through recovery. No matter how small." — Warren, 31, Ontario, Canada

"I focus on the positive way of thinking. When I was entrapped with all the shame and guilt, I found it impossible to look at the positives. I no longer dwell on the bad; I look for the good. I can understand that I am not the only person who was hurt. I am fighting back. I will become an advocate for the sexually abused after my pursuit of justice is completed." — Dennis, 50, Illinois

"...the present and future, recognizing that the past is just that — past." — Greg, 39, Indiana

"...my future, which at one point, I did not have or think of..." — Jim, 24, County Strathclyde, Scotland

Most of all, in great numbers, men write triumphantly of their ability to use the past differently, *let go* of its hold, and focus on *the present*.

"...to use the past experience as a device for gaining strength and knowledge instead of it being a focus of failure or discontent. I can now focus on my family and life in general in a new lightened and spiritual manner, which I could not do before." — Jeff, 43, Nova Scotia, Canada

"...strengths and challenges, the 'Now-ness of my life'...positive aspects of my life....solitude time." — Tony, 32, South Dakota

"...living in the present..." — Jon, 53, Kentucky

"...my *current* experiences." — Bob, 39, New York

"...the 'HERE AND NOW' through positive self-affirmations and planning healthy, realistic goals..." — Mark, 34, West Virginia

"...living in the moment — the here and now." — Al, 21, Ontario, Canada

"...structure...pay[ing] attention to the symbolic and work a day experiences in...life because they can really act as flags to inner process." — John, 33, County Devon, England

"...solutions and living in the present. The effects of my abuse still manifest themselves by sometimes restraining my forward movement. I have to push myself in order not to get complacent and to be satisfied with the progress I have made." — Bill, 49, Michigan

"...taking my experience (the pain, anger, and courage) and living day by day and sometimes minute by minute. I acknowledge what I survived and use to get through the rest." — Dale, 42, Hawaii

And more and more and more. And so much more.

"Today, after many years of hard work and therapy, I am finally learning to thrive, not just survive. As a matter of fact, I consider myself a thriver, not a survivor.... Life through recovering from incest is at times frustrating...but today I wouldn't trade that healthy frustration for a million dollars. It is so good to feel life (I numbed it for years with booze and drugs). I have been out of therapy and in recovery for five years and enjoying life. The horrors of the incest and physical torture don't come every night anymore, and when they do come, they aren't as bad and they don't stay around for as long...I now know how to deal with it all. And, oh, yes, they still hurt so bad, but I know it won't last. Both my wife and myself are survivors/thrivers, and boy did we experience some serious insanity in our travels through therapy. But we are so much stronger now that we have survived and defeated an enemy that has claimed so much innocence. As a matter of fact (again), a lot of survivors who know our story look up to us as a guideline to a healthy relationship. Don't get me wrong, we still have our moments of ugliness because of our individual incest problems, but we don't create wreckage and we solve our problems...."

May God continue to shine His grace on you." — [part of a letter from] **John, 38, Oklahoma**

It's hard for me to believe that anyone could read the quotes in the preceding pages and remain unconvinced about the reality of recovery. Creativity, power and generosity of spirit shine through statement after statement. They speak for themselves, but they also speak for all humanity. The next section features men speaking directly to their fellows.

Part Four

VICTORIOUS MESSAGES

— MAN TO MAN —

ARGENTINA TO ZIMBABWE

Some years ago, I was in Sacramento, California, conducting a professional training on male survivor issues. I had been bemoaning the inadequacy of the words that are most commonly used in recovery. I complained about the limitations of terms like *victim* and *survivor*, the somewhat stilted feeling of the word *thriver*, the robotic tone of *AMAC* (Adults Molested as Children), as well as the impossibility of referring to someone as a *liver*. After listening politely to my whining about the lack of a good term for individuals who have achieved their recovery goals, a woman in the back of the room stood up and suggested, "How about 'VICTORS'?"

Yes! That one felt right to me. After all, isn't it victory that we are after? Victory over the injuries of childhood; victory over messages of discouragement, blame, and shame; victory over hopelessness and despair; victory to live lives that are whole and healthy; victory to experience joy. Victory! Victors! Victims no longer. Now, Victors. Yes, it works for me.

I thank Debbie from the Sacramento training for suggesting this splendid word.

The fourth question on the Request for Resources form provides an opportunity for male survivors to speak directly to one another — man to man, survivor to survivor, thriver to thriver, victor to victor. I continued adding to this section even after I had finished the rest of the manuscript, because I kept on receiving important contributions.

Question 4 is:

"Something I would like to say to other male survivors is..."

The responses are amazing. Men reach out to their brother survivors, powerfully and profoundly offering support, encouragement,
advice, experience, wisdom, and love. There is a wide range of
response, from therapeutic to poetic, literary to scientific, analytical to
emotional, practical to visionary. Some sentiments appear again and
again. When this occurs, I will include several examples, since I believe
that important truths are worth repeating. These statements have the
ring of truth, because they are the result of genuine experience. I hope
that you, the reader, will accept these messages as guideposts and affirmations on your own road to victory. You may choose to use them like
vitamin pills — reading one each day. (If you do it that way, there is
more than a year's worth contained here.) Take time to really listen to
these words and feel the love they contain.

Alejandro, 27, Argentina
There is nothing written in Spanish for men who were abused. The
code of machismo does not permit understanding. I pray that the
changes you are making in North America will one day help to create
progress in my country.

Jose, 41, Argentina
I have hope that the situation will improve. It is good to know that
there are other men such as I. To know that you exist gives strength to
me. Thank you.

Mauro, 47, Argentina
We are on a shared journey

Doug, 37, New South Wales, Australia
Believe that you can become stronger through facing the past and
dealing with it. Like replanting a farm ravaged by a storm, it takes
patience, hard work and lots of care. But in time — as you deal with
yourself lovingly and nurture yourself with compassion and understanding — you will grow and flourish.

Eric, 29, New South Wales, Australia
Weep and scream — get in touch with your own pain.

Gordon, 57, New South Wales, Australia
Never give up hope. Be kind to yourself. Learn to love yourself at
whatever stage you are at — because you are special.

Danny, 25, Queensland, Australia

Mixed feelings abounded when I spoke of my trauma to my family. It was hard for them to accept that I was hurt and harder again that I accused an older male relative. Shunned somewhat by my immediate family, I found refuge with my new family; my close friends and partner who have supported me and given me comfort. Without them I don't believe I would have been a survivor.

Paddy, 49, Queensland, Australia

Courage

What courage to endure
To pay so dearly
For undelivered and unknown goods.

What patience to wait
For times of peace
So far out of sight.

What strength to hold to life
Than to relax in huge fatigue
And slip into the arms of nothingness...

David, 49, South Australia, Australia

Find a support group and a professional, *encouraging* counsellor. If men can disclose to their family and a few trusted friends, it helps reduce the loneliness and isolation. (My abuser was not a family member.) Cry as much as you need to and don't push yourself too much. Try to start liking yourself — it wasn't your fault that while you were a boy you were betrayed by a trusted adult. I eventually found the strength to take civil action against my perpetrator, not for revenge but to make him accountable. I confronted him with the support and presence of my psychologist and solicitor. This was terrifying to begin with, but there was a huge relief as the meeting progressed. It helped reduce the "power" he had over me and also reduced the guilt and shame which has consumed me for thirty-seven years.

Andrew, 27, Victoria, Australia

When all you can see is a blizzard, and all you can hear is the wind, there is no ground beneath to feel, and your soul feels stretched so thin you are wholly transparent — remember you are there, still there, and ultimately you are inviolate. You are beautiful. Your spirit is strong.

Christopher, 33, Victoria, Australia

No matter how pathetic and lost you feel, your quality of life is enhanced with understanding of where you come from, and that your future is yours to mould. The power is within.

Johny, 39, Victoria, Australia

In the final analysis, our journey sees us become something greater than we ever could have been without the wounds — that caused us to take the journey.

Neville, 58, Victoria, Australia

There is no gain without pain. You must accept that you will experience many forms of emotional and psychological pain in the process of healing from childhood sexual abuse. It is a long, rough, painful journey, BUT YOU CAN HEAL. I have. Remember the little boy that you once were. He was a survivor — a tough, resilient little Man. Don't quit. He didn't.

Patrick, 42, Victoria, Australia

When you were young, your own special and precious pearl with the whole image of you shining on it was thrown away, and now by finding many new and rich experiences or pearls from helpers, the jigsaw will piece by piece knit back your own special pearl yet again, as you never give up finding it, nor forsake hope.

Richard, 26, Victoria, Australia

Opening up to others and telling them of the sexual abuse has given me a path. I couldn't find the way on my own — I needed and still need, the help of others.

Sam, 36, Victoria, Australia

Find the strength within, and remember to tell yourself you are not the victim.

Tarran, 42, Victoria, Australia

You are not going crazy; it may seem and feel like it, but, sorry to tell, I don't think you are. Each of us is unique; we all react to trauma in different ways. Your reaction to what has happened to you as a child is YOUR normal reaction to an abnormal situation. Sexual abuse to me feels like the closest thing I ever went through to next to dying. And I almost have died, so I know what I'm on about there.

You cannot change the past, only your present, and your future. If you can, think of life as a journey, but it is something that is worthwhile to do. Giving in to suicide is only giving the abuser the ultimate in violation, domination, and victory. Self-injury and self-social destruction is perpetuation of abuse. It is, however, something that is tied to our image of self and our self-worth. Think of this if you can: give way to the fury and lash out at those you love and you only eventually hurt yourself. No one else. That, too, is perpetuating abuse on a different level, in a different way. Do you choose to willingly do that? I think that no one would. Stop and think. Learn to manage your fury; learn to stop and smell the roses when stress hits.

Alcohol and other substances work in the short term, but not the long term. Multiple relationships can satisfy one need and never another. Respect yourself and your partner. Listen to the breath between the words where nothing is heard but something is felt. Get to know who and what you are. You will find that you are not an object after all; you are a humane human being — your rapist was not. Be sensitive to the needs of those that care and love you. No experience that you have been through justifies harming another human being.

Travis, 28, Victoria, Australia
Try not to procrastinate and try not to be afraid and be ready for anything.

Markus, 31, Austria
There is nothing to be embarassed about or ashamed of. You have survived against enormous difficulties, and you are healing in spite of enormous pain.

Scott, 43, Brazil
Sexual child abuse is little recognized or talked about in Brazil. There is one survivor group in Brazil — in Rio — which is very far from where I live.... Five of them (women) came to visit me here...and we held my first survivors' meeting in my room. It was a very powerful experience for me.... [ML — Scott's statement is evidence that no matter how isolated you think you are, there are always resources available. Keeping looking for them. Keep insisting on them.]

Mik, 40, Grand Cayman, British West Indies
Holding, touching, and working with clay is a great way to connect with buried feelings.

Mark, 34, Alberta, Canada
Do not let the traditional values that society has of men confine what and who you are.... The healing process is multifaceted...a long journey filled with pain but also, and more importantly, great joy.... At this point in your life you are, for the first time, responsible for both.... The person that abused you took away the past, not the future — the future is truly yours.... You have survived. Now it is your time to prosper.

Brad, 35, British Columbia, Canada
Enough is enough. Do whatever it takes to break the cycle. Find the inner strength to accept the unfortunate past for what it is...*the Past.* Take the time to heal a little bit today. You are worth it.

Geoff, 27, British Columbia, Canada
My little guy applauds you and so do I.

Gordon, 45, British Columbia, Canada
...Imagine you have gone into the attic of your house and found a box for a thousand-piece jigsaw puzzle, and the picture for the puzzle is mostly gone from the front of the box. When you open the box, there are only one hundred pieces there. You start doing the puzzle and you find other pieces strewn around the attic. As you put more pieces together a picture starts to emerge, and you feel you know what the finished puzzle will look like. But a few more pieces make you revise your idea. You realize you will not know the way the puzzle will look until you get it totally completed. And no one else can tell you you what the completed puzzle will look like...as your puzzle is unique. It is up to you to keep searching for the pieces of the puzzle if you want to view the entire picture. When you get fed up [with] looking for the pieces and ask, "Why am I doing this?" You realize that the picture is of you and that is the reason to keep working on it.

Patrick, 64, Manitoba, Canada
You need the support of other male victims of one or another form of childhood abuse.

Ram, 50, Manitoba, Canada
[You] need to talk and speak out so that others may seek help and not feel alone in their fear and shame of being sexually abused.

Daniel, 39, New Brunswick & Ontario, Canada
There is hope in recovery, even though it might be hard. You are struggling with confusion, suicidal thoughts, low self-esteem. You can see yourself through if you want to — if you work hard at it.
Shop around for a good therapist.

Pierre, 28, New Brunswick, Canada
We do not have many resources for men, but we are the only ones who can do something about it — hand in hand with everyone who has been affected — direct and indirect victims, male or female. Let's build what has not yet been built and become conquerors instead of meekly accepting survival.

Robert, 47, New Brunswick, Canada
Open yourself a little more. Feel the challenge. Feel!

John, 32, Newfoundland, Canada
Go for it! Fully! Wholly! Passionately! You are worth life and love and health and strength. Settle for nothing less. Recovery is possible, likely, in fact, if you want it, if you work for it, and if you demand it. I have found a life beyond anything that I would ever dream of, and if it has happened to me — in northern and isolated Canada — it can happen to you. Fight for your healing. Take back your life. Come, be part of a whole new generation of men!

George, 43, Nova Scotia, Canada
Believe that — despite what happened — you can make your life different. And, with support, a tremendous amount is possible.

Jeff, 43, Nova Scotia, Canada
Find someone you can trust to talk to — someone who has been abused or a good counsellor. Someone you consider your best friend may not understand your problems in full. Group counselling is very good. Don't be discouraged if you are feeling down after after several months of admitting abuse, because it takes time to heal. But it will get better with time.

Jerry, 47, Nova Scotia, Canada
It is a long and painful process, but there is a light at the end of the tunnel.

Al, 21, Ontario, Canada
Don't run. Face the fear.

Barry, 38, Ontario, Canada
Tell someone! There is more help out there than you realize.

Bob, 46, Ontario, Canada
There is hope. It's okay to feel.

Dan, 34, Ontario, Canada
Invictus
Out of the night that covers me,
Black as the pit from pole to pole,
I thank whatever gods may be
For my unconquerable soul.

In the fell clutch of circumstance
I have not winced nor cried aloud.
Under the bludgeonings of chance
My head is bloody, but unbow'd.

Beyond this place of wrath and tears
Looms but the Horror of the shade,
And yet the menace of the years
Finds and shall find me unafraid.

It matters not how strait the gate,
How charged with punishments the scroll,
I am the master of my fate:
I am the captain of my soul.
           — William Ernest Henley (1849-1903)

David, 29, Ontario, Canada
Never, never, never, never, never, never give up.

Gregory, 37, Ontario, Canada
Never lose the child you once were. Keep part of him — that part may surprise you [with] how really strong it can be.... The one you

should be in touch with is you.... I wish you the best of luck on the
road to recovery. You will find it...a road to discovery as well.

Ken, 44, Ontario, Canada
You are not crazy! Celebrate your courage and strength and
resourcefulness. My heart joins with you, my brother, and we walk
beside each other out of the pain.

Marco, 31, Ontario, Canada
The day will come when you will notice the beauty of a sunset again.
When that day comes, be sure to congratulate yourself, as I did. You
have survived and there will be many more beautiful sunsets to come.

Murray, 41, Ontario, Canada
There is tremendous hope. Our pain is terrible and frightening, but
recovery is able to bring us to a new and wonderful life that, in a
pre-recovery state, we can hardly imagine.

Red, 39, Ontario, Canada
It was not YOUR fault. You didn't ask for it — [it] was forced upon
you.

Ron, 32, Ontario, Canada
Reach out to important, understanding people from your past and
risk talking to your best friend of today. Get involved in a good support group meeting weekly.

Sid, 33, Ontario, Canada
Abuse creates tremendous alienation and isolation — which makes
matters worse. Lots of effort is needed to connect with others.
Healing can only take place with the help of others.

Warren, 31, Ontario, Canada
The positive changes that I am now seeing in my life are worth all
the pain that I have gone through and all the struggles yet to come.

You are worth the effort that recovery takes and you deserve the
benefits that recovery has to offer.

It hurts, I know, But it IS worth it.

Mike, 37, Prince Edward Island, Canada
We alone are the only ones who truly know the right thing to do
about our own abuse.

Charles, 42, Quebec, Canada

Expressing the anger and rage will put you on the path to healing all the wounds.

Keith, 31, Quebec, Canada

A message I...have for others who are on this journey of recovery/rediscovery is not to rush. I heal of my pain only when I am ready and strong enough to uncover it, and not before.

Donald, 40, Saskatchewan, Canada

I'm so very glad you are recovering from incest. God bless you and grant you success.

Kristian, 52, Saskatchewan, Canada

YOU ARE NOT ALONE! Admitting that you have been sexually abused and victimized may be the most agonizing thing you've ever felt, but — in my experience — *knowing* that those were the facts of my childhood was fully worth that painful effort of acceptance. I would not return to my previous state of ignorance for anything. So much of my life that had previously been confusing and which had sent me into such inexplicable rages now makes sense. For me, that sense meant the lifting of a huge burden that had been oppressing me. It literally gave me a personal freedom and a basic "lightness of being" that have carried me through the subsequent rough times and difficult steps.

Luis, 35, Colombia

God bless you.

Luis, 22, Costa Rica

When we stand together, we will be victorious.

Douglas, 45, Czech Republic

Face the black hole and get whatever support you can in doing so.

Hamid, 52, Denmark

I will continue my own process; hopefully it will be not too turbulent. I have a kind of inner optimism. There will be ups and downs. The more I can accept what my childhood really was like, the better the inner quality of my life will become.

Jens, 31, Denmark

Stand free in the light of your own power.

Daniel, 39, Dominican Republic
Take care of your body, your health, and your spirit.

Jacob, 28, Dominican Republic
It is hard to tell the truth, but we must tell what happened if we are to survive.

Ali, 53, Egypt
Some days I wish that change would come faster. Yet I know that for a tree to grow takes time — to sink deep roots — to spread strong branches. Have patience. You, too, will grow stronger.

Billy, 42, County Avon, England
Connect with others in truth and love.

Joe, 50, Derbyshire, England
It's time to stop pushing people away.... Time to start trusting...loving in a truly intimate way, and time to start considering yourself worthy of life's greatest and simplest joys and treasures.

Bill, 36, Devonshire, England
Feel compassion for yourself and find the strength to continue with your own recovery.

John, 33, Devonshire, England
At many times throughout my recovery, it has felt as if I was robbed of the opportunity to live a normal life at the age of seven. I have heard this from many male survivors (and female survivors come to that!). Survivorhood is very useful in that it can provide us with a language and a sense that we are not alone. There is another side to it, however, which can be very seductive. Given this understanding and acceptance we can feel like it's the best we've ever had (and sometimes this is even true!). I want to say however that there is a danger here of living life like a war veteran hanging onto an event and living one's life in the shadow of that. What I want to say is this...grow out of it, then move on. Life is for living not surviving! I wish you well — Hang in there.

Paul, 43, Devonshire, England
Learn to love yourself, and direct your anger where it truly belongs.

A.H., 33, Leicestershire, England
Never give up hope, because despite the isolation we experience, often for many years, there are thousands — even millions — of us out there. It's perhaps easier to walk away and try to ignore it (that's what men are supposed to do after all!) But sometimes when we're lucky enough to find someone to trust and share our greatest fears with, something amazing seems to take place. It can feel like being reborn in the most liberating way I've ever experienced, perhaps a little like I imagine learning to fly might feel? Along the way, we make mistakes and do and say things that we might regret, but no journey was ever that easy, was it? Above all, be good to yourself. And with time you, too, will start to believe that you deserve to shake free those painful shackles and begin to realise that just anything is possible. Right now I really do think that it is.

Tony, 46, Leicestershire, England
Accept yourself and through that you will feel accepted by others, not as a man who was abused, but as a man in your own right. Do not be afraid of speaking about being abused; there are survivors everywhere. If you cannot do it alone, then join with others and have a voice. With others the road to recovery can be less difficult, though it may not seem so at the time. With others you can regain your self-esteem, your power, and your life.

Learn to love yourself; you are worth caring about. The pain may not lessen for some time, but the journey is worth making.

Duncan, 47, Suffolk, England
If, as I am, you are a corporal punishment survivor and have difficulty as an adult in consequence, then you probably find most adults, even professionals, deny corporal punishment as sexual abuse was once denied. Don't let this discourage you. Corporal punishment is wrong; it is abuse and your frustration, anger, and outrage are quite appropriate.

Michael, 43, Surrey, England
Always remember that [being] abused as a child...was *not* your fault. Release your anger in a positive way, either through a form of counselling that you feel comfortable with — or simply talk, shout, and cry with a friend you can trust. The more open you become, the greater

your self-healing process will work. One day you will learn to love yourself again and become that innocent, wonderful child you once were. Remember, it is never too late to have a happy childhood.

Olli, 38, Finland
We must end the silence of hidden crimes against children.

Hubert, 39, France
Care for yourself and hold to your dreams.

Luc, 52, France
They taught us pain and death. Now we must learn life and health.

Ingo, 31, Germany
Gebe niemals auf! Gebe niemals die Träume Deines Lebens auf. Du findest den Weg Dir zu erfüllen. (Never give up! Never abandon your life's dreams. You will find a way to fulfill them.)

Hartmut, 46, Germany
There is no other way of getting over it than feeling the whole hurt again that's been done to you.

Johann, 33, Germany
Good luck with your long-time work.

Jürgen, 36, Germany
All is not lost. There is a lot for which to live.

Thomas, 45, Germany
We must build a worldwide community.

Christos, 59, Greece
Let your fear lead you to courage.
Let your pain lead you to strength.
Let your sadness lead you to joy.
Let your darkness lead you to light.

Jean-Batiste, 40, Haiti
My dear friends. I celebrate your success.

Julian, 30, Hong Kong
The more I open myself, the more I feel refreshed.

Ashok, 45, India
Let the courage of survivors everywhere inspire you as it has inspired me.

Ramesh, 40, India
Have courage. Be strong.

Satish, 58, India
I wish you all you wish yourself.

Joe, 52, Ireland
Although it is so hard to break the different layers of silence, the effort and each success brings a life reborn (or rebirthing).

Kevin, 30, Ireland
Despite all the gloom, you will feel a happiness bubbling inside you — a kind of calmness about your life. Rest and have some fun. Play.

Michael, 28, Ireland
As soon as you are able to — cry. When I finally let go the tears in me, I finally released the little lad inside me. It was a cathartic experience.

Avi, 25, Israel
You have the right to exist. You have the right to belong.

Angelo, 58, Italy
Do it. The roads are many, yet there is no road: Just Jump!

Paolo, 40, Italy
We continue to struggle against the desire to be alone. I encourage you to continue your work. I hope for the best for all of us.

Matsuo, 21, Japan
Life is beautiful.

Teishiro, 34, Japan
Poetry is in your heart. Express your deep feeling.

Daoud, 46, Jordan
Let no one convince you that what you have suffered is unreal or unimportant. You must insist on your right to heal. It is difficult, I know, but it is vital.

J.V., 28, Kenya
You are my brothers and we are responsible for each other.

Ismail, 40, Malaysia
Have no shame for your tears. You have the right to them. You have earned them.

Alberto, 27, Mexico
Thank you for your brave efforts.

Hector, 58, Mexico
Recovering is a marathon, not a sprint. Even after running some miles, there is a long way to go. At the end, there is victory.

Sergio, 51, Mexico
Transformation is not possible until you face the truth. Then speak the truth from your heart and your soul.

Henk, 32, Netherlands
Face these experiences and slowly share them with your loved ones.

Joop, 54, Netherlands
Begin to think of yourself not as "surviving," but as "living."

Max, 50, Netherlands
Seek your happiness. Settle for nothing less.

Wim, 28, Netherlands
Together we are ending abuse forever.

Jehan, 37, New Zealand
You are not alone, and like our grandfathers and fathers before us, who faced their fears and had their bodies broken from Gallipoli to Normandy during the wars, we, too, face our fears and change humanity.

Ken, 45, New Zealand
.Share your feelings. Share your life. I found the major start to my healing was to share what happened to me, to give up the secret I had kept for thirty-three years.

Les, 60, New Zealand
It's not too late. You are never too old to grow.

Richard, 42, New Zealand
It is very important to be with other men who have gone through similar ordeals, to be able to talk about and share them.

Sam, 31, Nigeria
Now I can recognize a safe place when I am in one. So can you.

Svein, 60, Norway
NEVER GIVE IN. WE ARE OUR OWN EXPERT. We know what happened to us. We know the facts. We are not the only one. We are [a] very, very large population on this globe. And in the end, our version will [have] success due to all we have lost and might lose during our healing/recovery process — [No matter] how tough and dark the situation seems to be. Do not give in, because around the corner — the next day — a new day starts.

Mohammed, 42, Pakistan
Don't forget.

Carlos, 47, Peru
I am confident that the work we do today will protect young boys in the future.

Ramon, 36, Philippines
There were times when I wanted the pain to end and I almost gave up. I am happy that I did not. Someone came along and listened to me and believed. When you are afraid that you will not survive, and nobody in the world will understand your pain, please do not give up. Someone will appear to listen and to help. I am thinking of you.

Ryszard, 22, Poland
I send to you my friendship.

Bill, 40, Scotland
Be good to yourself and look after yourself.

Jim, 24, Scotland
Never give up, and if you feel trapped, get out. You can go on in life without being used all the time.

Peter, 43, South Africa
I wish you the best support, acknowledgment, and reconciliation.

Stefan, 51, South Africa
No matter how far apart we live, we are on the road together.

Juan, 67, Spain
You are a child of God. You are always in my prayers.

Magnus, 37, Sweden
We can set ourselves free to thrive.

Martin, 55, Sweden
It took nine years, but now I can be sexual and be joyful about it.

Klaus, 56, Switzerland
Accept the challenge to feel.

Kemal, 48, Turkey
You are not alone anymore. Wherever in the world you travel, there is someone who will understand you. You may not recognize him easily, but if you look and listen you will know him.

Anatoly, 49, Ukraine
Change requires hard work. I was challenged to think in different ways about my life. Good luck to you all.

United States:

Timothy, 37, Alabama
While the pain for me hasn't gone away entirely, it has become infinitely more workable. Still have difficulties with PTSD [Post-Traumatic Stress Disorder] and dissociative issues, but better and better. Still scary, but OK, too, in a weird sort of way. Life is good. The war is over. Take time out to go to the woods. Chop wood. Wax the car. Cook dinners with patience. Lean into the Silence and see what it has to say.

Bill, 38, Alaska
I feel safest among trees. Healing myself among our brothers the trees sprouts inside me a hope reborn of my whole humanity, my healed sexual self, my reconnectedness with my earth energy. My most profound healing happens when I am alone among the safety of all the great spirit's creations.

Will, 55, Arkansas
I'm getting better. Life is worth living. You can do it, too.

Frank, 57, Arizona
Don't wear the shame.
You're not to blame.

Gabriel, 22, Arizona
Like the Earth and Sky, you are holy. Learn to love your Sacred Self.

Treetop, 40, Arizona
For a long time, I was held captive in a dark and lonely woods by people who feared and hated the beautiful and loving child I was. Today I celebrate the wonders of my life from the treetops.

William, 46, Arizona
"It has come to my recent attention that witnessing a miracle can profoundly affect one's life. I encourage each and every one of you to join me in this experience. Gentlemen, step up to the mirror."

I spoke these words one day to my men's group shortly after approaching the Catholic Church for assistance.

Bob, 43, California
Don't feel guilty about what happened; You are not at fault. Don't try to do this alone. It's too big a load for one or even two or three people to shoulder alone. Let *all* your friends help, and remember to thank them.

Bob, 45, California
Do not let shame and self-destructive behaviors isolate and abuse you further. Find support and lots of it. Do not give up on yourselves.

Colin, 33, California
You did nothing wrong.

Dale, 45, California
Find a photo of yourself taken just prior to the start of the abuse, one where you are still happy, smiling, and full of life. Have it enlarged and hang it where you'll see it often. (Seeing photos taken of me during the years of the abuse are also helpful in my healing.)

Doug, 33, California
YOU ARE *NOT* ALONE! I spent many years feeling like I was the only man who had ever been molested as a child. I saw so many

resources available to women survivors, but few that seemed to be aimed at men. My advice to male survivors is to reach out into some support group, either on-line in CompuServe or on the Internet, or at a twelve-step meeting like SIA. There are other male survivors and there is support; you don't have to struggle with this alone.

Doug, 35, California
Realize that you are strong and find your inner strength. It's there. It's the thing that has kept you going all these years. It is both a talent and a gift.

Doug, 57, California
Find the spirit within, the wounded child within and pray for the courage to do the recovery and healing.

Gary, 46, California
Talk about it! We've lived in our dark rooms long enough. See the door. It's hard to open all the way. The door is heavy and the hinges are rusty. But you will pass through it!

Gene, 32, California
The best way to get over the pain is to slowly but confidently walk *through* it, and reverse the balance of power.

Jim, 46, California
Use art as a way of making your story concrete. Draw out the scenes of the abuse, and they will seem more real.

Pete, 30, California
Take care of your physical health! Stress, depression, and repressed anger can take a big toll on you!

Randy, 35, California
It's not that you are defective, but you had things happen to you that you survived.

Robert, 46, California
Never give up hope — even obsessions and terror can be transformed. You can find the good kind of peace.

Stephen, 34, California
Anything that would help make peace with a slow, slow, deep, and hard process.

Tino, 41, California
Beware of the victim trap. To brand yourself as a victim is to give your power away and it means that someone else still has control over you. Every time you say "I can't" because of what happened to you, your molester wins. Healing comes from expanding your self-view, and shedding the shame and guilt that are associated with victimhood.

David, 54, Colorado
In some ways, my life got harder before it got better. I had to own up, get honest, learn to feel and see how I had defended myself against anger, pain, grief, and fear. But while they've increased, so has my ability to relax, pay attention, let go, and get real. I'm beginning to discover my own power over the old demons which used to run my life from behind a facade. The less the facade, the more the honesty, the more grace strikes and supports my journey.

Geoffrey, 32, Colorado
I would encourage other male survivors to do whatever it takes to keep themselves out of denial. It would be great if I had never been sexually abused, but there is no more pretending. My goal is to continue to integrate this knowledge of my past into my current awareness of my being, without getting stuck on the abuse itself. I will always be a man who *was* sexually abused as a boy by my father's buddy. With conscious knowledge of this today, I make myself clean, whole, and proud to be male.

Steve, 50, Colorado
You do not need to relive bad experiences and relive bad feelings; it is not healthy for you and it is unhealthy for the ones you love. You need to acknowledge that you have had bad experiences, but you do not have to let those acts in the past govern your life in the future. By bringing abuse out into the open to even one person who cares and listens, you will realize that you are not alone anymore. I am proud to know you as a fellow survivor.

Van, 41, Colorado
My partner, John, and I are raising three healthy, confident sons. Life is full of good surprises.

Joel, 34, Connecticut
You are a shining star in the Universe.

Kevin, 39, Connecticut
Whatever numbness techniques you used to survive, you owe it to the child in you (and yourself) to cast them aside and get on with the healing!

Tim, 32, Connecticut
As bad as you may feel about yourself, there is a wonderful, caring person buried under the pain. You can release him by slowly letting in the love of others who are not hurtful. Having him in your life will make the struggle worthwhile, because he will *always* be there for you.

Wayne, 60, Connecticut
It may seem like it is taking forever, but you can get through the effects of the abuse by giving the shame back to your abusers.

Bill, 45, Delaware
My message to others is to learn to be committed to helping yourself heal. It takes a long time — not a short period of time. So commitment to one's self has been my salvation. Second, a support network to help and assist during the "process." It has to be one you create or find, but you must trust that they will be there for you.

Bob, 65, Delaware
Hold the hand of a friend or hold your own hand as you feel pain on the way and stick with the pain. Incredibly, only good results.

Bob, 68, Delaware
Start recovery now. It is never too late. It is never too soon.

John, 58, Washington, D.C.
Hang in there! It is a journey, and I'm awfully glad I'm on it with you and others just like us. Sometimes, when the next step seems too hard, I'll wash the dishes, or make the bed. With action I begin to participate with you again, and that's where I'm finding my recovery. *Welcome aboard!*

Paul, 34, Washington, D.C.
Something I would like to share with other survivors is my definition of recovery. It is being honest with *ourselves* about what has actually happened to us in our lives. If we can reach, and maintain,

that level of honesty with ourselves, then we can create the lives we were born with the right to live. Lives full of challenges and personal growth, but free from the negative effects of brutal, undeserved sexual child abuse.

Male survivors are some of the strongest, smartest, bravest, and most creative people on this planet. Surviving the abuse to be where we are now is proof of our strength, inherent wisdom, courage, and creativity. By working toward honestly sharing what has happened to us, and what we have learned, we can be all the heroes our children will ever need.

Allan, 40, Florida

When accessing and confronting the feelings and emotions, remember that the feelings [and] emotions cannot hurt you any more than you've already been hurt. Unleashing the Pandora's box of feelings related to the events is liberating, as it makes those feelings/emotions powerless over you.

Brad, 43, Florida

You are not responsible for your abuse.

Brendan, 48, Florida

Talk about it, talk about it — whenever, wherever, however. Only by breaking the silence can we heal.

Chris, 45, Florida

It wasn't your fault! You are not alone. Please join us in our quest to put a total and permanent end to male sexual abuse.

Jim, 37, Florida

You are *not* alone. There are tens of thousands of us out there who have experienced terrors similar to yours. Who have felt feelings similar to yours. You demonstrate your courage, intelligence, and toughness just by still being here. God bless you all.

Joe, 56, Florida

Pay attention to the old thoughts in your head.

Mickey, 52, Florida

Your strength lies in your relationship with a power greater than yourself! Be it church, AA, or a trauma clinic, God speaks to us through these people! God may also speak to us through the next song we hear, the next sentence we read, the very next person we talk to, so we must strive to stay in tune with the spirit of the Universe if we are to be not only a survivor, but a winner also!

Mike, 60, Florida
I was incested by my mother.... In my fifties I started to deal with it.... To others I would say: Find a support group. My therapist helped to form a gay men's group, and the six of us meet weekly to talk and talk and talk...and it really helped.

Roger, 44, Florida
Learn all you can about the consequences of the abuse. The abuse is not our fault, but recovery is our responsibility. Good luck.

Tony, 38, Florida
Take a step back to visit the past so you can move on with your life — and remember it's not your fault!!!

Val, 30, Florida
You have power!

Walter, 45, Florida
One of my greatest difficulties in healing from abuse was coming to terms with the senselessness of it all. One day, I realized that what I'd really wanted was to find someone who would make it all better, someone who would hold and comfort me and make me feel loved without feeling molested. But I was too old to crawl back into my mother's lap, and too suspicious of everyone else. I realized that the only way I would ever feel better was for me to find something bigger than me, something I could trust forever and ever. For me, it wasn't God because, as far as I was concerned, God had abandoned me when I needed him most. I had to find something else. I tried all sorts of spiritual journeys, but, ultimately, it was something wonderful from my childhood that brought me through: the ocean. Maybe the ocean will take me to God some day.

If there is anything in your childhood that made you feel better — a forest, the mountains, a corn field, a thunderstorm — go find it and be with it and take your strength from it. Then it won't matter if nothing else makes sense.

Benn, 32, Georgia

Take your time! It took a while to get this far, it's going to take a while to heal.... Take time for YOU. BUY A TEDDY BEAR! or a MOOSE or a DUCK or a...at 3 A.M. when you need to cry it out and are scared and it doesn't make sense, a bear WILL listen, and absorb your tears and sobs, and keep you warm and safe. Chocolate IS the fifth food group, eat it once a week, or take a bubble bath, or just do something silly and fun for YOU. (Blowing bubbles with the dog is my relaxer). YOU ARE NOT ALONE. I believe you. You don't have to live your life afraid of them. They were wrong. NOT you.

Kurt, 39, Georgia

My experience taught me that my rage and fear would always control me until I visualized them as a part of me and something that I could love and respect. These feelings will never disappear, but you *can* make peace with them.

Marc, 51, Georgia

...the process is long, but do not give up *your* hope. I can sincerely say that every step forward is one that you never retrace when you either fall down or backward. The recovery process is ongoing and our growth is never ending. The age of the adult and the age of that little boy inside so rarely coincide, but I encourage you to bond with him and love him. He will continue to share his secrets and his love. It is genuine love...as genuine as the abuse. Allow him to heal because your growth is defined by his growth.

Ross, 30, Georgia

Follow your heart.

Dale, 42, Hawaii

Find and get all the hugs and touching you can tolerate.... Don't stay physically isolated when all you really want to do is touch and be touched. Please *trust!* Trust your process, your experience, your body, and the universe — it does provide a way to face the hungry dogs behind the basement door. And please — *just being willing* even to just entertain the thought of a change in behavior is *so* liberating. Like opening an old cellar and letting in fresh air and light!

Rand, 38, Hawaii
Let your tears fall.

Frank, 37, Idaho
No more victims. No more survivors. Just people. We can make it happen.

Ray, 34, Idaho
You can do it!!

Rob, 33, Idaho
We all make a difference.

Bob, 48, Illinois
Forgiveness is *not* a recovery issue, anger is. Forgiveness is a spiritual issue, as is love, and both will come naturally after all blocks to them are removed. Over and over, I needed to blast God with my anger and then God simply began to fill that resulting void with love and peace. In an environment of love and peace, forgiveness grows naturally of itself.

Carey, 50, Illinois
Remember your three T's — Things Take Time even for me. Do your work and never quit.

Charles, 45, Illinois
You have the right to heal. There is help available. You can find a support network. Recovery takes time but it is worth it. Do this for yourself.

Dennis, 50, Illinois
Don't ever give up! It takes time, take a rest when you feel you can't go on. Don't rush into things; don't do things until you are comfortable with what you are going to do.... I promise you, the shame, the guilt, the dirty feelings will go away if you work for this. Surround yourself with supportive people; avoid negative people. Try to think positively; do not take on other people's problems. Be supportive of others in recovery. Give them support only when you can.... Without jeopardizing your health...painful and difficult decisions must be made by you and for you. *Is it worth it? YES!* Define your boundaries ...respect others and demand to treated respectfully, too.... You will find support from some of the least expected places.

Henry, 30, Illinois
I have found myself healing faster once I accepted the fact that the recovery process is just that, a process; it will not end the way the need for it began — in an abrupt, single event. This has allowed me to replace the anxiety and panic my self-imposed time frames for "getting better" evoked with the positive feelings of hope and trust that I will get well.

Iceman, 20, Illinois
Recovery sucks, but it's worth it!

Jack, 48, Illinois
Life to me is about attitude. If you tell yourself that it sucks, then surely it will. But if you tell yourself that it is wonderful, it surely will be wonderful.

John, 29, Illinois
Reclaim your life. Don't let "trying to figure out why it happened" keep you from moving forward. There may not be an answer. Just know that it shouldn't have happened, that you didn't deserve it, and that what's important now is to get it behind you, love yourself, and grow!

Bernie, 49, Indiana
The work is hard, but well worth the work.

Greg, 39, Indiana
God has always put "angels in my path" in the form of strangers, friends, family, and counselors. Listen and look very carefully. You are not, never were, and never will be completely alone. [ML — In a letter to me, Greg added the following:] ...when I speak of angels — I don't mean heavenly spirits with wings and halos — I mean ordinary people. Looking back, whenever I was at my absolute lowest, a person who [would] say something, do something, be somewhere.... Always these things seemed coincidental and insignificant at the time — but they weren't. Too many "coincidences" happening at just the "right time"...I wish for you the "insight" to recognize the angels in your path, too.

Mark, 30, Indiana
Don't be afraid to face the fear that is deep within. Healing and cleansing come from getting it out. Also, consider telling others

about [the] abuse when you are ready. The abuse uses the victimizing power of silence.

Patrick, 55, Indiana

There is HOPE if you are willing to look at your pains and to acknowledge your hurts. Rather than trying to pretend to be normal, find a safe place to share your feelings and to learn to value yourself. Survivors are loving and caring people who have much to offer others.

Stan, 47, Indiana

Your natural instinct is to be apart from. Reach out and be part of.

Matt, 20, Iowa

Believe in your dreams.

Osvaldo, 41, Iowa

Your goodness is and always has been within you. Lastly, and something that was somehow important for *me* to hear as I recovered, is that I am very sorry your childhood was in any way painful for you. Here goes a hug.

CC, 45, Kansas

Read Mike Lew's book *Victims No Longer*. Eradicate the hate for your abuser(s) from your system. Hate is vicious [and] eats its host from the inside out. Find a way to vent your anger in a safe way.... Develop assertive thinking. Refuse to be a victim any longer. If you...choose a mate, choose a supportive one who understands.

Jim, 58, Kansas

When I found other male survivors, the world became less lonely. I am glad you are out there. I am here for you, too.

Eston, 43, Kentucky

Find the Divine energy within you and worship it. It is perfect and undamaged.

Phillip, 48, Kentucky

Learn all you can about this and don't isolate yourselves.

Charlie, 41, Louisiana

Take all the time you need.

Mark, 30, Louisiana
You're not alone. Find support. Work [the] twelve steps. Reach inside of yourself and get the anger, hurt, fear, and the tears out in a positive way. Learn to feel the feelings again.

Jim, 35, Maine
Pain is frightening and agonizing. The good part is that it changes. You can always count on that, if you do your work. Looking inside is excruciating — it also frees you. The emotions and events of early and mid-recovery felt devastating to me, and I was convinced I could never survive them. It's good to be wrong sometimes — it's great to appreciate my own humanity.

Tom, 61, Maine
You never deserved what happened to you.

Bob, 43, Maryland
Never give up hope — to give up hope is to be dead.

Bob, 75.6, Maryland
Reach for the time — long or short or never in this life — when forgiveness is possible.

Jim, 32, Maryland
Don't let fear stop you from asking for what you need or want. Asking can be absolutely terrifying, and it takes tremendous courage, but the rewards are infinitely fulfilling!

John, 43, Maryland
Hang in there.

John, 61, Maryland
Finding people that I could trust and opening up my deepest thoughts to them has brought my spirit back to some level of fullness. I feel, I care, I am more involved.

I believe that this festering must be treated with honesty and truth and openness. Only then can a survivor begin the needed growth to become who he should have been his whole life.

May God give a special blessing to all of His survivors! This is my prayer.

Mike, 51, Maryland
Talk. Talk. Talk. Talk about the sexual abuse and what it did to you and then talk some more. Keeping it all inside only adds to the burden, slams the door shut on the only way out.

Adrian, 45, Massachusetts
The road to recovery is a long and hard path to follow. However, if you believe in a God, either internal or external, he gave us a potential, and it is our duty now to fulfill that potential — despite or because of what other people may have done to us.

As survivors we must do everything possible to repair any damage that we may have done to others starting with our immediate partners and children. We must stop the toxic cycle passing on from generation to generation.

Ajith, 43, Massachusetts
One day, I found out that "Everything I ever believed was wrong."

Angelo, 25, Massachusetts
Recovery is a process, not an event. It may take time, but recovery is a reality. I have gone through a lot of pain and legitimate suffering in order to heal. There is nothing like the joy of recovering yourself.

Bill, 47, Massachusetts
You are not alone, and your recovery must not happen in isolation. You went through the abuse alone — your recovery must not.

Charlie, 37, Massachusetts
Take time for yourself, no matter how hard it is to carve that time in your daily life; you need lots of time to reflect, exercise, and feel all the feelings. Listen to and respect your feelings, positive and negative; they are valid and worthy.

Dan, 28, Massachusetts
Don't ever give up. Remember that you are a good person and what happened was not your fault (not our fault). It's OK to love yourself. There are more of us out here ready, willing, and able to help.

Dave, 52, Massachusetts
Progress seems nonexistent until I look back a year ago.

de Pietro, 34, Massachusetts

You are strong. You have both inner strength and outer strength. Strength enough to protect the part of your being that is still a child. Say to that child, "I love you. I will protect you. Do not fear. Do not doubt. I am with you always; I am your protector and your strength."

Jim, 26, Massachusetts

Give yourself a break and remember that the abuse happened in the past. It doesn't have to continue now and in the future by beating yourself up for it. I spent untold numbers of hours, days, years telling myself I was crazy, messed up, or not good enough. Not only was it not true, it was further from the truth than I could imagine.

As I continued to press myself to feel, I realized that while sometimes I might have a different view of the world than "normal" people (whatever that means), that often times my special view was insightful and is quite often creative and useful...my views and thoughts really did matter and I didn't need to give any more power to those lying messages from the past.

John, 36, Massachusetts

The Healing Road

Come along friend
and walk with me awhile;
I see your load is heavy
and I'll help you if I can.

How long have you been wandering, lost
and alone in this dark grove?
Did you hear the drumbeat
of your brothers' marching

and glimpse the light
of our torches through the mist?
It was eighteen years
before I found the Healing Road

and I've been marching now
for five.
Gonna find that bright horizon, man.
Gonna find that pot of gold.

Before we get old,
we're gonna find it if we can.
As long as we're alive,
and as much as we allow

ourselves to unload
our pain and fears, our rage and tears,
to raise a fist
and beat back the relentless night,

we can keep marching.
Through numbing cold and blistering heat,
we strove
to get here, beyond the holocaust.

Now, just a little farther in this sad caravan;
I know it's just across that burning levee
by the Styx, and we're gonna smile. We're gonna smile
in the end.

John, 49, Massachusetts

Use your wisdom when you are most rational to put in place a system which will help you when you are least rational. Be both persistent and patient with yourself. It probably took a long time to arrive at your current condition, so expect it also to take a long time to get better, but do expect to get better.

John, 52, Massachusetts

Recovery *is* possible.

Ken, 51, Massachusetts

Don't be afraid to admit/acknowledge what was done to you. Be assured that you're not alone, that many others have suffered and experienced the devastating effects of the abuse; that while some of your reactions, feelings and actions may not seem "normal," they are very normal for an abused person. Read as much as you can on the subject and seek the help you need individually and with others.

Kenny, 41, Massachusetts

Your guard can come down and your soul can be free to love again. The abuse can not and must not define you.

Michael, 42, Massachusetts
The human spirit is strong and resilient. It can grow and transcend any hurts with the right support from other people and the right caring and self-accepting attitude by the survivor. Always remember that you are much more than the abuse and you have a great potential to share with others. Above all, none of the abuse is your fault.

Moe, 63, Massachusetts
Trust your instincts, your experience, a good therapist, and God being there for you.

Oliver, 53, Massachusetts
The pain of my early sexual beginnings will not go away, but it becomes more bearable by sharing it with appropriate people. I no longer have any secrets — someone else (not necessarily just one person) knows as much about me as I do about myself. Knowing that I'm not alone and that I'm not defective is bringing me more and more to feeling that I'm part of the Human Race.

I now have the opportunity to live a more full, more happy, whole and holy life as I journey on this wonderful (yes, painful) road of self-knowledge, self-love, and love and acceptance of others.

I'm on the road — one day at a time.

Peter, 37, Massachusetts
You're not alone in this world. Reach out to us — we're here; we support each other.

Richard, 45, Massachusetts
I have come to the following belief — that there is no past but this incarnate consequence I call "myself" — and I am not, and none of us are, done changing.

Rick, 47, Massachusetts
Joy is worth working for and waiting for; structure your own recovery as feels safest and most comfortable for you; don't buy into other people's agendas no matter how compelling they might seem. Your first responsibility is to yourself: Take care of yourself, be both an adult and a child, be the best parent to yourself that you can be.

As incest victims we learned to accept abuse as normal, and the imprint of that abuse is hard to shake off. Though we may find it hard to imagine and accept that we are worthy of joy and pleasure in life, we are. We deserve the best and we don't have to act like our perpetrators to get our needs met. They were sick people and we reject their sickness as we move into living life and reaping its positive rewards.

Rick, 51, Massachusetts

A critical part of my recovery was making "the connection," the understanding that much of my undesirable behavior is a direct response to someone else's intrinsic flaws, and not a reflection of my true self. Making the connection continues to be a grounding that facilitates my ongoing progress. Remember to make the connection!

Sean, 29, Massachusetts

Despite how overwhelming the pain may feel today, it will pass, and you will feel relief. The healing process takes a long time — be very patient! Once you have thoroughly worked through your sexual abuse issues, you will be more powerful and more alive than you ever imagined. You will not only be a survivor, but a thriver!

Stephen, 51, Massachusetts

Then: I felt as though I had gone so far away from myself that I would never be able to come back or even want to. Never mind knowing how.

Now: Through all the fear, shame and pain which has held me in a prison, not of my making, but of those who raped me of my innocence as a child.

With the support and encouragement of a therapist and, most profoundly, the safe love, support, and encouragement of other male survivors, I am on my way back to a place I never could have dreamed of — a safe place within.

Bill, 49, Michigan

Keep on trying. Keep on working and working at this healing process. We must continue to break the silence or it will keep coming back to us. We must also continue to work with others to help empower them to learn freedom and happiness our recovery brings.

David, 61, Michigan

Seek help. Only now is it clear that what I lacked was help because I didn't think I needed it...that I came through with a sense of humor, I hope is evidence of courage, and perhaps a little genius.

Frederick, 54, Michigan
Pray to the god of patience, and ask for it, for healing is *SLOW.*

Jim, 55, Michigan
Resources for recovery are available but not well organized nor well publicized. Seek out other survivors in your area and find out about proven resources for male survivors, including psychotherapists, psychiatrists if medication is indicated, variety of male support groups, variety of weekend workshops, and medical professionals experienced with survivors. Organize your own program for recovery. Seek advice from other survivors and professionals who are experienced with the healing processes of survivors. Be sure to include spirituality as a component of your healing to provide the foundation of goodness and hope which is needed to face the terror, despair, rage, and grief that are inevitable parts of the healing journey. And most of all remember there are many, many male survivors. *YOU ARE NOT ALONE.*

Scott, 41, Michigan
Allow time to pass in order to heal and gain an objective view along with the sometimes oppressive subjective view.

Ted, 26, Michigan
Believe!!! If you embrace the light of Recovery, you will be delivered from the dark pit which you have lived in.

Tom, 40, Michigan
Learn all you can, and be steadfast in your commitment to recovery, but always be gentle with yourself. You ARE deserving of love — including your own.

Alford, 55, Minnesota
The comfort of one's fellows sustains. Hang in there! Love your inner child!

Ed, 46, Minnesota
Hurt and pain are part of every life. There are those with whom you may find empathy. Do not be afraid. But be honest with yourself, and to the extent you feel safe, be honest with and demand honesty from others.

Jon, 47, Minnesota

"Recovery" and "healing" mean you are going to grow in such a way that you can put your childhood into a context you can understand and accept. "Recovery" and "healing" also involve letting go of some things, perhaps even some long-held hopes or dreams....

Other people can give you encouragement and hope, but you are the only one who can do the intense, difficult work of growing and healing...it will become less and less necessary to keep bringing up old, troubling memories, allowing you to spend more time looking ahead and less time looking over your shoulder....

As you heal, your friends and family who, knowingly or not, have suffered along with you, heal along with you.

You cannot heal by yourself, and you won't heal until you're ready. When you're ready to heal, you'll find the strength to reach out and get the help you'll need....

Your personal healing will be speeded and strengthened if you simultaneously work to heal your community, dedicating yourself in whatever small way possible to ensure that what happened to you will not happen to another child.... In a way, you're an expert.

Derek, 29, Mississippi

You are worth it!...worth the trouble and pain involved in the arduous task of recovery. This is not your fault and you are strong enough to stand up to this task. Ironically, in time, after much pain and tears, you will understand what Melody Beattie means when she says, "It will be better than you ever imagined," because it will be.

This journey cannot be started alone. Involve a trusted therapist and do not forget about the love, compassion, and grace available from your Higher Power and the still, small voice inside of you.

Jimmy, 23, Mississippi

I didn't think it was possible to get my life back. If I can do it, so can you.

Ron, 52, Missouri

You are not alone in pain, fear, anger, confusion in your will to live. There are those of us who have been and are presently sharing the horrible pain. I don't know you personally, but I feel we are bonded by strengths greater than we can imagine. You are held in the utmost safety of my heart...always!!

Geoff, 50, Montana

There is help through truth, vulnerability, and making healthy choices. I found health seeking/living men and women critical to my recovery. I found healing through looking at similarities rather than differences. I was able to find my own spirituality through others by feeling the joy and pain and through acceptance of unconditional love from others.

Rick, 35, Montana

Don't go it alone. Find someone you can talk to and share your thoughts and, more importantly, your feelings.

Rodger, 31, Montana

I commend them.

Bill, 40, Nebraska

There can be life in recovery. Don't give up yourself any longer. You are a beautiful, valuable human being who is stronger than anything that has happened to you. Live YOUR life!!

Bo, 56, Nebraska

The cycle stops here. My children will never go through what I did.

Pat, 42, Nebraska

There is Hope.	Don't give up Hoping.
There is Love.	Don't give up Loving.
There is Happiness.	Don't give up on Life.
You can make it.	Don't give up on Yourself.

Tony, 44, Nevada

Reach out, Brother. Take my hand. We can do it together!

Ben, 32, New Hampshire

We are not our abusers. We cannot and should not let their actions against us dictate the kind of life we should lead. We don't have to fall into the traps that they set for themselves. We can rise above our victimization and take control of our lives. We survived the most horrible thing that can happen to any person; we can face and surmount anything else that life throws at us.

Jim, 42, New Hampshire
Never stop asking for help. You may have negative experiences with family, friends, therapists, doctors, lawyers, policemen, but never, never stop asking for help! The enemy is withdrawal and isolation.

Also, Jack Kennedy once said, "There are only three things that are real: God, human folly, and laughter. The first two are beyond our control, so it is best to focus on the latter." I whole-soul agree!

Steven, 26, New Hampshire
There is someone out there that accepts you as is — not what they want you to be — but as *is*!

Barrett, 40, New Jersey
"This ain't no party — this ain't no disco — this ain't no foolin' around."

Chris, 21, New Jersey
Each time you take a risky step and express what you feel, you discover who you really are...divine and love. You are perfect.

Fred, 20, New Jersey
There is hope, and one day when I have...conquered this, I will look back at a survivor who is just starting and say, "Remember, no matter how hard it may seem, know it can only get better. So just hold on and REMEMBER THE LIGHT AT THE END OF THE TUNNEL IS YOU."

Michael, 40, New Jersey
Everything that I lost or thought I lost is coming back to me as I find the courage to keep in the open that which has been kept in the dark for so long.

Rick, 41, New Jersey
Discovering a hobby helped balance the "work." The first male survivors workshop felt as if I'd safely come home, just as group psychodrama enabled me to understand I'd been struggling to become what I already was — human.

Tom, 40, New Jersey
Recovery from abuse is a difficult process. For me, the effects of the abuse have taken time, coming off one layer at a time, so to speak.

But every bit of the process has been worthwhile, providing me with more and more freedom and joy with life as each layer is healed. It is amazing to me that the area of sexual identity and attraction can and has been part of this process. I am grateful for each and every step of my healing process.

Zandy, 44, New Jersey

I'd encourage you to find your medium, e.g., dance (for me), in a safe environment to give yourself/selves the opportunity to begin speaking. Our subconscious mind's needs get met in safe ways — illuminating our conscious minds — as we begin to say, "Ah ha" or "That's why I do this" or " I know who's talking now and why." I guess I'm saying we're worth it. Let's find our safe medium and grow through this stuff.

Aaron, 29, New Mexico

Throw out that macho mentality because it will kill you! Take help. Strength is having the courage to feel those terrible and good feelings. Feelings won't kill you.

David, 57, New Mexico

We survived this terrible tragedy called our "childhood." We had the strength of will, the courage to do it, and we need, at rock bottom, to honor ourselves for surviving a very hostile culture.... I think we need to speak out for today's children and the children of the future....We all need to support each other.

Bob, 39, New York

The first thing that came to mind is "Don't give up!"..."Take care of yourself." That is my advice, hope, and prayer.

While being abused, we took care of ourselves. Period. We may have done it by forgetting, by playing make-believe, by leaving our bodies, by participating, by smiling and laughing, by finding reasons why this was happening to us, by blaming ourselves or any combination of the many just and creative ways we came up with to survive at the time. And we did it. Damn, we are resourceful. Be proud of that victory.

Repression, denial, food, or whatever worked then, can work today. When your fix-it doesn't work anymore, maybe it means everything is OK and it is time to cast and sling things aside.

Be the doctor you always needed. Take care of yourself.... Do not give up. Don't let the bad people win. Love, Dr. Bob.

Bob, 45, New York

Believe it, trust in yourself, disregard others' criticisms, trust in yourself, feel the pain. If it needs to be done — do it, even if it's painful or uncomfortable. [A] joyful, Good Life.

Chris, 50, New York

I always thought that the sequelae of childhood sexual abuse would kill me, probably sooner than later...intractable suicidality, chronic depression, writing and reading paralysis — but they did not. As I broke my silence, they became the things that validated what I had been through and helped me to see that my life was not a pathetic exercise in self-execution, but rather a source of inspiration for myself and many other people.

Clain, 38, New York

Hugs, Kisses, Cookies, and Ice Cream.

Daniel, 36, New York

We need to see the beauty in life to survive. Search for beauty early in your healing, if only for a moment, and find beauty in a line you draw, a lyric, a lost emotion, or even a blade of grass.

David J, 42, New York

Once you have identified yourself as a survivor and seek recovery, one of the *greatest* resources of support, growth, and keeping a positive attitude is to find at least *one* and *as many as possible* people who are recovering as well — that you feel some connection to. When two or more meet and share, the whole abuse cycle is broken. Over and over again.

Don, 50, New York

This is the hardest work you may ever do, and will be the most rewarding work of your life. It has been for me. You will get your life back. You are not alone. You have my love and respect.

Donal, 41, New York

Find other men who are survivors. We need each other. Be gentle and patient with them and yourself. It will be scary. In fact, it will be excruciatingly terrifying and painful. But the rewards are bountiful. All the years of frozen energy used so carefully to keep the pain away, will be unlocked. Our innate abilities for loving kindness will be our greatest gift to ourselves and to those in our lives we wish to share intimacy with. Ah! The taste of true intimacy will be savored in your soul forever.

Doug, 46, New York
The abuse never goes away — only the way we think about it, and in that is redemption.

Doug, 46, New York [another forty-six-year-old Doug]
For me, taking anger out in a safe and appropriate manner was — and will continue to be — defining.

Doug, 48, New York
Stop blaming yourself. Stop trying to hurt yourself. One day at a time, you're not defective.

Frank, 34, New York
We are, unfortunately, many. You are not alone. Seek out those who can play a part in the healing. Step by step, I've tried to come into the light. So far, it feels warmer here.

Gary, 32, New York
"There's a hero — if you look inside your heart.
You don't have to be afraid of what you are.
There's an answer if you reach into your soul,
and the sorrow that you know — will melt away."
— Mariah Carey.

Hanibal, 39, New York
Keep fighting and confronting your past until the feelings become memories.

Ira, 44, New York
Don't give up. Notice the little beams of light that stir you. They help show the way along the dark path.

James, 45, New York
Inside are the tools of strength and courage to chip away at this painful obstacle — to finally be free and alive — to live in peace and love myself.

John, 24, New York
When I have the urge to numb out, escape, return to addiction, withdraw, or not take care of myself, I imagine all the people who abused me lined up in a row, cackling at me — a piercing and sobering reminder that, when I honor myself, the abusers have no power over my new life. In short: LIVING WELL IS THE BEST REVENGE.

John, 30, New York
It's possible to recover to love and trust again.

Joseph, 62, New York
Talk to a safe person(s) — Believe your story — Get help in a twelve-step program — get therapy from a therapist trained in abuse. Trust God.

Larry, 32, New York
Page 83 [of] the Big Book of AA...The "Promises" of AA are helpful.

Larry, 35, New York
I try to live my life like the Prayer of Saint Francis. I try not to harm others and myself and practice balance.

Lawrence, 35, New York
It gets much better if you just stay with it.

Lawrence, 62, New York
Many, many thanks for being here; trust the growing network of comrades who respect "touching by invitation only," and affirm our right to speak and be welcome...we can rejoin the creative magical child...the wonders of our childhoods are not lost.

Lloyd, 44, New York
Transformation is possible — healing is *real* and remains with you.

Michael, 31, New York
SURVIVE. Whatever it takes. Because while we've seen that life can hold a hell of a lot of pain and anguish, it can also...offer a wondrous amount of love and happiness. We've been through the worst; now we must seek the other, better side of things. It may take all of our imagination, our ingenuity, our intelligence, our strength, and our

patience, but we mustn't ever stop. Life is very important. And to have life, we must survive.

Michael, 42, New York
It's not true that men don't have feelings of fear, shame, guilt.

Paul, 41, New York
I am glad that I am a man. (This was not always so.)

Pete, 36, New York
Once you truly believe it is possible to heal, it starts to happen.

Pete, 49, New York
Finding out that you're not alone and being open to listening to other survivors can save a lot of pain.

Ralph, 29, New York
Be creative. Heal and Be Healed.

Rich, 30, New York
This whole process is worth it; you're worth it. I love you!

Stefano, 29, New York
Recovery and healing are possible for us. Trust in the process. You will experience great freedom!

Steven, 37, New York
You are not alone.

Todd, 32, New York
You are not alone. Many others have stories almost the same as yours.

Tohon, 35, New York
Seek to validate, whenever and wherever, what you already know to be true about the innate value and beauty of life. Don't give in to what J.D. Salinger would call "sloppy thinking."

Tom, 36, New York
From the SIA preamble, "You were not to blame, and you are not alone."

Tom, 59, New York
We are all very brave. To live with the fear, rage, and pain and still be here, still healing...We are very brave.

Vince, 33, New York
As a victim of sexual abuse...I sense that I am much more sensitive and in touch with my overall feelings.... This sensitivity, I believe, is one of my greatest strengths. It puts me at an advantage in maintaining my health and well-being as a male.... I am confident that in order to ensure success in my recovery, I need to continue honoring my sensitivity, while also learning how to protect my sensitive side when having to cope with toxic people.

Xandu the Giant, 33, New York
Break the silence and talk about your incest or sexual abuse victim experiences when/where you can. You'll *feel better* (eventually) and your healing will begin. Survivors' groups are a good source of support and understanding.

Some people will not want to hear your truth and will attempt to prevent you from speaking out — don't let these people stop your healing process; listen to your own true voice.

Always remember: DON'T LET THE BASTARDS GRIND YOU DOWN!!

Good Luck.

Anthony, 31, North Carolina
Healing requires allowing ourselves to hurt enough to embrace all the miracles hidden within our pain. Find that person out there who allows you to take down your wall long enough to experience a glimmer of healing. Then, before you know it, you'll take that wall down — brick by brick. Recovery is worth all the risks of fear, rejection, abandonment, and loneliness. We must flee the isolation that clothes all survivors and welcome the miracle of true intimate (not sexual) healthy relationships.

Don, 34, North Carolina
It is not your fault. The abuse was nothing you had control of, nor did you have the power to stop it. The responsibility for the abuse belongs to the abuser.

Michael, 46, North Carolina
Find the "right" therapist. Write in your journal. Find other men who have undergone abuse also.

Michael, 52, North Carolina
Define who you are and do *not* allow someone else to do it for you.

Rick, 35, North Carolina
Every time I express pain in a constructive way, it releases its hold on me a little more.

Roland the Recovery Beast, 29, North Carolina
You are a child of God, no less than the trees or the stars. You will recover. You deserve and are worthy of love and life.

Steve, 36, North Carolina
The road to recovery is lengthy and can be extremely painful. However, there *is help available* and you *can* recover. Remember that you only have to live in the present moment. Free yourself from the past and [be] present. Don't isolate yourself. Reach out for help. You don't have to be alone anymore.

Bob, 57, North Dakota
Don't be afraid to talk about the abuse. Be kind to yourself. You are only as sick as the secrets you keep. Be of service to others and live a day at a time.

Chris, 57, Ohio
Just by going through the process of facing the facts of what happened, and acknowledging I will probably never remember it all, feeling that pain and allowing that rage to truly be felt, has brought me to a place where there are actually glimpses of serenity in my life. During this process, I found ME, and I am learning to know him and love him.

Davis, 54, Ohio
We are not responsible for being abused, but we are responsible for our recovery — together and with anyone who loves us.

Michael, 30, Ohio
Be careful if you choose to expose your perpetrators either via the criminal or civil law systems.

Michael, 38, Ohio
That you are not alone, that abuse happens to boys more than anyone would care to admit, that there are networks and chat rooms and

groups of your brothers and sisters meeting somewhere near you right now. We must protect and defend one another, especially when men are first coming to grips with the impact of the abuse on their lives, when they are most vulnerable. In providing strength and support to one another, in protecting one another, we are creating a safe community in which we ourselves, the protectors, will also be protected.

Mike, 36, Ohio

Feel the feelings. As I uncover more uncomfortable, sometimes terrifying feelings inside of me associated with the abuse, it is essential for me to embrace them. They are like the little kid parts of me, wanting desperately to be heard and held — throw tantrums (raging, depression) if unacknowledged, and so relieved when I let them speak through my feelings. *And* Don't Give Up! You can get better — with the help of trusted friends.

Mike, 51, Ohio

Persevere, deepen spirituality, pray, connect more with that great source of faith, whatever you call it — God, Higher Power, Deepest Self.

Mike, 54, Ohio

Get a good therapist and trust him/her completely — find good meetings and attend faithfully — connect with real and supportive friends — pray as much as possible (it is the greatest source of personal strength) — take good care of your whole person regularly. The results will be: continued personal growth in recovery, learning and consciousness raising, deepened spirituality, learning a healthy self-care and self-love, and learning to share your gifts with others and to love them.

Rob, 38, Ohio

You are not alone. The problem was not you — it's what was done to you — and you survived beautifully.

Brent, 35, Oklahoma

You're not alone. Get help; it's out there.

John, 38, Oklahoma

We (your fellow survivors) are out there (real world). We know and understand so well what you're going through. Know that we care, read *Victims No Longer*, a truly amazing book for *us*!!

Kenneth, 49, Oklahoma

It's not a "little" thing.... It's not harmless.... A child's concept of self lives on in the adult's concept of self...Wrongful touching is no "little" thing.

Arthur, 65, Oregon

Take Heart!

Brian, 39, Oregon

Work on yourself. You can leave on a camping trip without preparation, but then you find yourself in the woods unprepared.

Clay, 24, Oregon

I'm movin' on.

David, 27, Oregon

Notice what's beautiful. It was always there, but pain clouded my view. Take another look.

Bob, 39, Pennsylvania

Keep on moving ahead. Don't be discouraged by setbacks.

Bob, 47, Pennsylvania

Your feelings do matter. Be gentle with yourself.

Chuck, 53, Pennsylvania

Don't stop working on your issues. Life gets a lot better.

Geoff, 35, Pennsylvania

Use a variety of resources. Read. Develop faith in a God of your choice — believe that you can't do it alone, and develop trust in others.

Gug, 46, Pennsylvania

I share your pain. I walk the road of recovery with you. I share your joy and new life.

Kevin, 35, Pennsylvania

Please don't judge yourself or your actions, past or present.... Accept that you're trying to heal the pain.... I'm learning to respond to love and let go of the abuse.

Jeffrey, 41, Pennsylvania

Healing comes...it is not easy. Trust the process. Put one foot in front of the other...and keep walking. You are worth it.

Larry, 44, Pennsylvania
Take care of yourself. You are good and worthwhile. Open up to others and to love. And keep yourself safe. Don't let anybody hurt you or use you. You are a beautiful guy.

Len, 50, Pennsylvania
You will find, as I have, that in your loneliest, most frightening, heartbreaking moments, you were sharing what most other abused men knew; this community of shared experience heals.

Owen, 51, Pennsylvania
Find a safe space/place to be unsafe in.

Paul, 36, Pennsylvania
Keep the faith, brothers; I need your support.

Tom, 44, Pennsylvania
You are not alone in having been abused, and you are not an impostor at life or a phony, although you're almost sure to feel that you are. Join a group of male survivors; seek out male survivors. There's comfort, help, and healing to be had with/by your fellow survivors.

Will, 37, Pennsylvania
The most difficult thing for me in surviving has been to separate the physiological response I had during the abuse — my own arousal — from the victimization.... For years I could not see myself as a young man who had been victimized because I had felt pleasure...my anger at this is something I am...now able to deal with...

Patrick, 35, Rhode Island
Read *Victims No Longer*. Get a good therapist....Arrest any addictions through going to the appropriate Anonymous Programs available. I recommend Co-dependents Anonymous wholeheartedly. Give yourself a break — and break your silence. Talk therapy works. Read *Knights without Armor* [by] Aaron Kipnis. And *King, Warrior, Magician, Lover* [by] Robert Moore and Douglas Gillette. These help solidify the ego and access emotion. Hold on and pray to all and any Gods — and let yourself heal. Remember, you are loved. And in my prayers. Your brother.

Patrick, 42, Rhode Island
Hang on. Hang in there. I'm with you.

Rod, 48, Rhode Island
When I first saw the title of *Victims No Longer*, I said, "Yeah, sure." But recovery really works. I'm not a victim anymore.

Alan, 32, South Carolina
Many men have found their way through the swamp to a bright new day. So can you.

William, 62, South Carolina
I used to be a survivor. Now I am thriving!

Erik, 47, South Dakota
Don't doubt your knowledge of the reality of the abuse, even if you are without all of the factual details. If you must have factual proof, examine the reality of the *effects* and the cause will be clear.

Fight the belief that your reactions are unique. For me the strength to take some of the hardest parts of my journey of recovery has come from the time spent with other survivors. From them I learned that my pain, grief, fears, experiences, worries, secrets, acting out, behavior patterns, and shame are NOT unique, but part of a normal and rational reaction formed in response to an incomprehensible situation.

The 20 percent of recovery that is the easiest concerns information. Knowledge about sexual abuse and its effects in general, and awareness about the abuse I experienced and the effects in my life is important. It gives me a framework of understanding. The 80 percent of recovery that is the hardest concerns activity. The actual change that has occurred in my life has not come from knowledge or understanding, but from changing my behavior—usually in small increments. I am learning to feel emotions rather than avoid them by some compulsion or other. I am learning to act in ways that are different than my historic patterns. Acting in new ways takes a lot of courage and consistency takes a lot of self-discipline. Usually I go two steps forward and one step back. But it has always been the action not the knowledge that has produced change in my life.

Steve, 42, South Dakota
Take the risk of sharing the reality of your life experiences — you will most likely be let down by some, however, this is the best way to find supportive people.

Tony, 32, South Dakota
Either give up now or move on. It Hurts Like Hell, but going through to the other side has been worth it for me. Make your own decisions....

Don't forget *Humor* — Gallows or otherwise!!

Happy, 47, Tennessee
Through therapy you can find the safety that you long for. Don't give up! Keep trying until you find the right therapist and the right group. It is the difference between life and death. You have been dead in your body long enough.

Randy, 36, Tennessee
Life isn't perfect, but it keeps on getting better.

Terry, 49, Tennessee
Keep trying. You'll get it someday.

Chris, 22, Texas
You're not alone. Even though no one has been through exactly what you may have been through, the recovery is all similar.... The process is not quick. The occurrences will never go away. But you can move on.... We are not abnormal. We have simply been through something that some men have not. Don't let it cripple your life.

Dwayne, 44, Texas
Don't give up. I thought about suicide. I even took sleeping pills to end all the hell. It's been four years since I was in hospital. With lots of ups and downs, and lots of crying time, I think a person can get through it....

I think it's very important to find a good counselor....

Things get better.

Jay, 40, Texas
Go to any length to learn your truth. Choose Life!

Joe Henry, 45, Texas
It's important to do the work (recovery). It's the hardest thing I've ever done...but living with myself...the pain...the suffering (is) was insufferable...have to do the work.

Ken, 53, Texas
Be gentle with yourself and trust the process. You will give yourself a precious gift.

Larry, 53, Texas
There's a lot of help out there. Get it for yourself. You deserve it.

Mike, 39, Texas
Before you're ready to share, become best friends with yourself and with God. When you become ready to share, find someone you can trust and share as regularly and meaningfully as you can.

Nick, 47, Texas
Accept the love and wisdom of survivors in recovery.

Tino, 25, Texas
We as survivors have each other to overcome our fears, insecurities, and memories. We can do this by supporting each other positively.

Blaine, 40, Utah
As a gay Mormon survivor I didn't think I had a chance...too many strikes...but I made it. Anything is possible.

Brent, 48, Utah
Nothing is more painful and frightening to me today, than to realize I could have gone to my grave shackled by the bondage of sexual abuse. Knowing that my soul had never come alive to experience being truly happy, joyous, and free. Today I SOAR with the eagles and embrace lovingly my very Soul. My twelve years of recovery have come as the result of "consistently going against my better judgment," of allowing God to lead me and coming to know intimately that the price for dignity is pain, and the price for true freedom is even more pain. "Short-term pain for long-term gain" daily reminds me to never ever stop this miracle of recovery. God wants me to have the very best of life and today *I agree with Him.*

Bill, 50, Vermont

I made it through the pain.

Olin, 42, Vermont

It never hurts worse than it already does.... Acknowledge to yourself how bad it was, how much suffering you endured. This makes it possible to *grok* what a strong, powerful man you must be to have endured that.... Trust your subconscious.... It's OK to do this work a little bit at a time, in two-ounce doses. You can put it on the shelf for a while and then come back to it. It won't go away until you are finished with it.... You do get finished with it.... You don't have to love your mother.... The only way out of the cycle for any of us is to deal with our own pain. We can't have compassion for others until we can have compassion for ourselves. And we can't have compassion for ourselves until we know the depths of the pain we have suffered.

Frank, 28, Virginia

You are not alone. There are others — other men — who have experienced feelings similar to your own. For many years I felt unique. Unique in my pain, anger, fear, hopelessness, and self-loathing. Suicide seemed like a real option for me during those years.

What I've come to know is that I am not unique. So many men have similar experiences to my own. How grateful, yet sad, I am not to be alone. And there is strength, love, and certainly hope in sharing experiences and feelings with other survivors. Life today is worth living. All the messages that previously led me to other conclusions were not my own messages. They were the messages that my abusers trained me to think and say to keep me from reclaiming my own power, strength, and goodness.

It's still sometimes difficult to weed out those negative, abusive tapes. It is and will be my lifelong journey. What gets me through the tough times is the knowledge and feeling that I am good — good to the core.

Talking and sharing experiences with other male survivors feeds and reinforces this central belief. Those same conversations also allow me to give back the negative messages to the abuser and, most importantly, to live. It's a struggle. It's a journey. And it's absolutely worth it.

Fred, 38, Virginia

Yes it hurts. Yes it is horrible. Yes you can grieve. You are not alone. Yes you can heal. Yes you are OK. Develop your faith.

Mitch, 40, Virginia

Healing yourself is your spiritual destiny and your gift to the Universe.

Mitch, 37, Virginia

Find one person who helps you laugh. Find one thing you enjoy doing and embrace it, hands first, then arms, body, and soul. Thank you Nicky, my angel.

Sam, 26, Virginia

Although your family of origin or others close to you may not believe or try to deny you, believe in yourself first. It is the first step in unlocking the pain. The rest will follow, including unknown strength and power. I believe in you and support you.

Brian, 19, Washington State

Look Deeply. Please remember yourself, remember how to smile, remember it's okay to love, it's okay to laugh and find happiness.

Gene, 59, Washington State

The abuse was not your fault, no matter what the circumstance. Be not ashamed and know you are not alone. Seek help and support as soon as possible. The residues of this terrible circumstance can be worked through and we can have a life better than ever. However, give yourself time. It is vital to learn to allow yourself to be loved by others and to focus on gaining trust in yourself — and then others. Risk loving back when you are able.

George, 61, Washington State

...just the word TIME. At the hospital, they had an equation written on the wall. It was:

$$\frac{\text{GRACE (Unconditional love)} + \text{TRUTH (honesty)}}{\text{TIME}} = \text{HEALING and FREEDOM}$$

Thor, 55, Washington State

Reach out, Brother. Take my hand. We will succeed together.

Mark B., 34, West Virginia

Please, please talk to someone, possibly a minister, pastor, or chaplain. Talk to even a total stranger if need be because, for me, I found the abuse didn't hold as much power and control over my life — as it had for so many years — once I had talked to someone. Just open your mouth and speak. Strangers in the fellowship of others is perfect, for the majority are there to help or be helped, so they have an ear to hear you! The road to recovery begins by taking this step of talking to *someone*! Just do it and let the healing begin!!

Warren, 25, West Virginia

You don't *have* to feel like shit forever.

Avoor, 48, Wisconsin

It may be difficult, long, unpredictable, but life is enjoyable; one should keep moving ahead.

Curt, 43, Wisconsin

Believe in yourself, always remember that it wasn't your fault. You *are* special and important; you can get through the pain, and you're not alone.

Roland, 56, Wisconsin

Keeping your feelings locked up takes a lot of energy. It drains you. When I stopped trying to keep it all in, amazing energy got released.

David, 35, Wyoming

If you can admit that you were sexually abused, then the rest will get easier as you go. Never give up, because if you do, then those who abused you will win and they will be able to control you for the rest of your life.

John, 43, Wales

You must keep on working at recovery. Do not quit; you are not, and never will be, alone. I would say that there are no better vehicles to move the recovery process forward than reading others' experiences and also writing about your own. However inept your writing skills, the truth, as the saying goes, will always out. At the end of the day, it must be your own feelings and intuitions that you listen to. The child within will know what he/she wants, even though the adult is not always listening. Trust yourself; believe yourself; love yourself. If you can, revisit the earlier days of your life and try to re-discover your innocence; find the child you were and bring that person home to safety.

Nigel, 44, Zimbabwe
Out of all the wrenching pain comes HOPE.

Afterword
HOW FAR WE'VE JOURNEYED AND WHAT IS AHEAD

We have come a long way from the days when isolation seemed the only available alternative to abuse — when survivors would suffer further abuse in adulthood because their loneliness had become too painful to bear. We've made tremendous progress over the past decade, but we're not yet home free. Many obstacles continue to challenge male survivors, their allies, and the recovery movement overall.

The backlash against survivors who stand up against abuse continues unabated. Memories are still labeled "false" because they are not precise or continuous. Therapists and counselors working with survivors are still accused of "instilling false memories" in their clients — for who knows what nefarious purpose. Most therapists I know would be more than happy not to have to deal with the painful issues of abuse and recovery. So would most survivors. The idea that recovery is just the latest fad or some sort of club that people can't wait to join is simply ludicrous. People go into recovery because they need to; it's too painful not to. They've tried everything else and the pain persists. No one decides to dredge up painful feelings and memories for the fun of it. To think otherwise shows how little some people understand about the long-term effects of abuse and the nature of the recovery process. Certain individuals and groups have reasons, personal or economic, for trying to keep survivors and their allies silent. Those who believe that counselors have the power to instill memories — even if they wanted to — demonstrate their lack of understanding of the strength of survivors.

But the attacks continue. Therapist-bashing is a popular (and often lucrative) sport among some reporters and lawyers. A number of the leading advocates for survivors, including Laura Davis, Ellen Bass, Renee Fredrickson, and David Calof have been subjected to vicious attacks, lies, character assassination, and frivolous, harassing lawsuits. Although they are frustrating, costly, and time-consuming, these attacks have not succeeded in their aims of silencing survivors, demonizing their therapists and stifling voices of healing. There are many dedicated, caring people within the legal system and mass media, but there are also unscrupulous individuals, eager to profit from pain. Be aware of the potential danger of being revictimized and retraumatized by a system that does not honor your needs. While compensation and restitution (and sometimes punishment) are possible through the legal system, there is no guarantee that you will be understood or that your needs will be respected. The legal process takes control over the timing, pacing, and intensity of recovery out of the survivor's hands. Be very careful if you choose to pursue legal action.

There are other problems facing male survivors and those who care about them. As in other fields, a number of professionals are trying to co-opt recovery, taking power away from survivors. Some individuals seek to establish a rigid professional hierarchy of abuse treatment, complete with licensing examinations, official organizations, approved courses, and other manifestations of self-seeking careerism. Be suspicious of any so-called professionals who set themselves up as knowing what you need better than you do. Be particularly aware of people who would pathologize your recovery by taking a "healthier than thou" attitude.

Some people attempt to profit from the natural desire for a "quick fix" or "magical solution" by offering simplistic formulas or marketing gimmickry, "one size fits all" techniques. Whether in the form of books, therapeutic techniques, or recovery programs, it is important to be wary of easy answers to complex questions. No one has the right or the knowledge to tell you what you *must* do about your own healing. Your recovery consists of a series of courageous acts. And, in a wonderful line (from a recent film whose title I can't recall), "One should always be brave in one's own terms, and not anyone else's."

There are those who continue to belittle the issues of male survivors. Even now, men who were abused as children may encounter ridicule, contempt, dismissal, denial, and minimization. While this is less frequent, it should *never* happen.

There still are attempts to keep survivors separated from their natural allies, producing isolation that would keep them weak. This sabotage takes many forms: criticism of individuals or groups, creating false distinctions, playing on fears and doubts, fomenting racism, sexism, homophobia, heterophobia, ageism and other damaging "isms," encouraging misunderstanding, stereotyping and jealousy. When we replace the isolating reaction of "I'm jealous" with the healthier response of "I admire" or "I'm interested," a number of benefits result. We open ourselves to different views of reality, and become better able to effect meaningful change in our lives through our own efforts. We learn the vital lesson of accepting mistakes and imperfections in others; by extension we become more forgiving of ourselves. No one is perfect; we have all made mistakes and will make more. What is important is not perfection, but admitting our errors, learning from them, making amends where possible, and committing ourselves to not repeating the same mistakes.

Yes, there are lots of obstacles. We still encounter toxic, vengeful, and jealous people. Children are still abused and not enough is being done about it. The effects of abuse are not taken seriously enough by families, communities, governments, or helping professionals. There needs to be far greater funding of prevention programs, education of professionals, informing the general public, and treatment of child victims and adult survivors. This is especially true for poor people who require access to resources that are available to wealthier individuals. It is true for people of color, who have ample reasons for suspicion of agendas imposed by outsiders who don't understand their cultures and values. Opportunities must be provided for minority communities to educate their own members, creating services consistent with the values of the group.

We need far greater recognition of the difficulties experienced by survivors' spouses, partners, and other loved ones so that supportive resources can be developed. We need and deserve more services of all kinds, whether provided by the government, professionals, or survivors themselves.

Male survivors need more and more connections — with one another, with female survivors, and with other allies. This is coming to pass. As is evident from the responses in this book, male survivors are learning that human connections are crucial. In the words of one recovery joke:

Q. How many male survivors does it take to change a lightbulb?
A. You can do it all by yourself, but it's OK to ask for help and support.

Male survivors are also learning that their recovery is not dependent on anyone else's behavior (and certainly not of the ones who abused them). They are giving up unreasonable expectations of their partners, therapists, friends, and family. By letting go of impossible hopes and demands, they open the door to healthy, meaningful relationships.

There is ample evidence that male survivors (with significant help from female survivors and other allies) have made important progress over the years. I doubt that it would have been possible ten years ago for films that address male survivor issues (such as the excellent and heart-wrenching *The Boys of St. Vincent*) to be made, let alone distributed in theaters and video stores. We did not see major sports figures like star hockey player Sheldon Kennedy and Olympic gold-medalist diver Greg Louganis speaking out about having been abused — and being taken seriously — or baseball superstar Mark McGwire donating three million dollars to the fight against child abuse. Books by noncelebrities, like Richard Hoffman's *Half the House*, would not have found a mainstream publisher — nor would a major television network have picked up his story for a prime-time program. (On June 20, 1997, *Dateline NBC* aired a feature on the book and its effect; the show was remarkably free of exploitation.) A decade ago, churches, schools, and other institutions were not held accountable for abusive actions by their personnel; governments were far more likely to cover up sexual child abuse than provide programs to deal with it. We did not have nearly the number of books, articles, television and radio programs, films, and plays with male survivor themes that exist today. There were far fewer resources available for survivors or being developed by groups of male survivors themselves.

The men who shared their experiences in this book made a number of things abundantly clear. They state, lucidly and forcefully, that recovery work produces changes that are real, important, and permanent. They have made a commitment — to themselves and to one another — to doing whatever is necessary to put an end to cycles of abuse. They show us what has worked for them, and inspire their fellows to remain steadfast on their own healing paths. They have come to respect their own pace and level of intensity, letting themselves off the hook, and encouraging you to do the same. They demonstrate, again and again, their intelligence, creativity, bravery, perseverance, vulnerability, strength, tenderness, insight, and caring. They have learned to love and offer their love to all of us. They let it be known that not only do we need one another, we *have* one another. They are proclaiming victory over sexual child abuse. They are heroes; they are brilliant. They are leaping upon the mountains and skipping upon the hills. And they are inviting you to join in the dance.

Resources

RESOURCE BIBLIOGRAPHY

This is a list of the books and authors cited in response to the questions in the Request for Resources, or otherwise recommended by male survivors. Wherever possible I have included full titles and publication information, sometimes with my comments or those of the men who recommended them.

Allison, Dorothy
1992 *Bastard Out of Carolina*. New York: Dutton. (A powerfully written novel by a powerful woman. It carries the honesty of experience.)

Andrews, John
1994 *Not Like Dad: One Man's Story of Recovery from Incest*. Toronto: Macmillan Canada. (A courageous personal history by a Canadian survivor.)

Bass, Ellen, and Laura Davis
1988 *The Courage to Heal: A Guide for Women Survivors of Child Sexual Abuse*. New York: HarperCollins. (The original "bible" for women survivors; it has also provided help and guidance to many men.)

Berendzen, Richard
1993 *Come Here: A Man Overcomes the Tragic Aftermath of Childhood Sexual Abuse*. New York: Villard Books.

Berry, Jason
1992 *Lead Us Not into Temptation: Catholic Priests and the Sexual Abuse of Children*. New York: Doubleday.

Black, Claudia
1990 *Double Duty: Dual Dynamics within the Chemically Dependent Home.* New York: Ballantine Books. (Claudia Black has written many helpful books for adult children of dysfunctional families.)

Blume, E. Sue
1990 *Secret Survivors: Uncovering Incest and Its Aftereffects in Women.* New York: Wiley.

Bradshaw, John
1988 *Healing the Shame That Binds You.* Pompano Beach, FL: Health Communications.

Chopich, Erika J.
1990 *Healing Your Aloneness: Finding Love and Wholeness through Your Inner Child.* San Francisco: Harper & Row.

Cleaver, Eldridge
1967 *Soul on Ice.* New York: McGraw-Hill. (An autobiography that made history by a man who influenced a generation.)

Colgrove, Melba, Harold Bloomfield, and Peter McWilliams
1976 *How to Survive the Loss of a Love.* New York: Bantam.

Corneau, Guy
1991 *Absent Fathers, Lost Sons: The Search for Masculine Identity.* New York: Shambhala (Random House).

Davis, Laura
1990 *The Courage to Heal Workbook: For Women and Men Survivors of Child Sexual Abuse.* New York: HarperCollins. (Laura Davis was very careful to be completely inclusive of men in her wonderful workbook.)

Engel, Beverly
1989 *The Right to Innocence: Healing the Trauma of Childhood Sexual Abuse.* New York: Jeremy P. Tarcher.

Farmer, Steven
1991 *The Wounded Male.* New York: Ballantine Books.

Forward, Susan, and Craig Buck
1978 *Betrayal of Innocence.* New York: Penguin.

Fossum, Merle
  1989 *Catching Fire.* (audiocassette) Minneapolis: Metacom, Inc.
  1986 *Facing Shame: Families in Recovery.* New York: W.W. Norton.

Fredrickson, Renee
  1992 *Repressed Memories: A Journey to Recovery from Sexual Abuse.* New York: Simon & Schuster. (An influential work that continues to be attacked by many who deny the validity of survivors' memories.)

Gannon, J. Patrick
  1989 *Soul Survivors: A New Beginning for Adults Abused as Children.* New York: Prentice Hall.

Gil, Eliana
  1983 *Outgrowing the Pain.* Walnut Creek, CA: Launch. (Eliana Gil's writing for survivors is clear, straightforward, and helpful.)

Graber, Ken
  1991 *Ghosts in the Bedroom: A Guide for Partners of Incest Survivors.* Deerfield Beach, FL: Health Communications.

Gurian, Michael
  1996 *The Wonder of Boys: What Parents, Mentors, and Educators Can Do to Shape Boys into Exceptional Men.* New York: Putnam.

Heller, Joseph
  1974 *Something Happened.* New York: Knopf.

Herman, Judith
  1992 *Trauma and Recovery.* New York: Basic Books. (This book is required reading for professionals who work with survivors.)

Hoffman, Richard
  1995 *Half the House: A Memoir.* New York: Harcourt Brace. (Every survivor, male and female, will benefit from reading this extraordinary work. So will anyone who cares about truth, honesty, the struggle for healing, reconciliation, and the ultimate triumph of right over wrong. For more of Richard Hoffman's writings, recorded interviews, and helpful links, see his Web site at http://www.abbington.com/hoffman/index.html.)

Hunter, Mic
1990 *Abused Boys: The Neglected Victims of Sexual Abuse.* Lexington, MA: Lexington Books. (In this and other books, Mic Hunter has done much to educate professionals about issues of male victimization.)

Janov, Arthur
1970 *The Primal Scream: Primal Therapy, the Cure for Neurosis.* New York: Putnam.

Keen, Sam
1991 *Fire in the Belly: On Being a Man.* New York: Bantam.

King, Neal
1995 *Speaking Our Truth: Voices of Courage and Healing for Male Survivors of Childhood Sexual Abuse.* New York: HarperCollins. (Further evidence of the courage and creativity of male survivors.)

Kipnis, Aaron R.
1992 *Knights Without Armor: A Practical Guide for Men in Quest of Masculine Soul.* New York: Putnam.

Lee, John H.
1993 *Facing the Fire: Experiencing and Expressing Anger Appropriately.* New York: Bantam.
1987 *The Flying Boy: Healing the Wounded Man.* Deerfield Beach, FL: Health Communications.

Lew, Mike
1990 *Victims No Longer: Men Recovering from Incest and Other Sexual Child Abuse.* New York: HarperCollins. (Originally published in hardcover in 1988. Outside the United States and Canada, it is available as a Cedar Edition of Heinemann Mandarin Publishers, London. The German translation is published by Kösel-Verlag GmbH & Co., Munich.)

Love, Patricia
1990 *The Emotional Incest Syndrome.* New York: Bantam Books.

Maltz, Wendy
1991 *The Sexual Healing Journey.* New York: HarperCollins. (A very accessible nuts-and-bolts book about repairing sexuality damaged by sexual abuse.)

McMullen, Richie J.
1990 *Male Rape: Breaking the Silence on the Last Taboo*. London: Gay Men's Press. (Distributed in the United States. by LPC/Inbook, Milford, CT.)

McNeill, John J.
1988 *Taking a Chance on God: Liberating Theology for Gays, Lesbians, and Their Lovers, Families and Friends*. Boston: Beacon Press.

Miller, Alice
1991 *Breaking Down the Walls of Silence: To Join the Waiting Child*. London: Virago Press.
1984 *Thou Shalt Not Be Aware*. New York: New American Library.
1983 *For Your Own Good*. New York: Farrar, Straus.
1981 *The Drama of the Gifted Child*. New York: Basic Books. (Alice Miller has long been one of the original — and finest — champions of survivors.)

Moore, Robert, and Douglas Gillette
1990 *King, Warrior, Magician, Lover: Rediscovering the Archetypes of the Mature Masculine*. San Francisco: Harper San Francisco.

Mura, David
1995 *Where the Body Meets Memory: An Odyssey of Race, Sexuality, and Identity*. New York: Anchor.
1987 *A Male Grief: Notes on Pornography and Addiction*. Minneapolis: Milkweed Editions (P.O. Box 3226, Minneapolis, MN 55403). (A brilliant poetic essay about the connection between sexual child abuse and adult addiction to pornography.)

Nouwen, Henri J. M.
1972 *The Wounded Healer: Ministry in Contemporary Society*. New York: Doubleday.

Peck, M. Scott
1985 *The Road Less Traveled*. New York: Simon & Schuster.

S., Joe
___ *Out of Hell*. (I was unable to locate any information about this work.)

Saint-Exupéry, Antoine de

1943 *The Little Prince* (Translation of *Le Petit Prince*). New York: Harcourt Brace Jovanovich. (This is the original "inner child" story. If you've read it before, try reading it again in the light of your current understanding. If you haven't yet read it, you're in for a special experience.)

Sanders, Timothy

1991 *Male Survivors: A 12-Step Program for Adult Male Survivors of Childhood Sexual Abuse.* Watsonville, CA: The Crossing Press. (Personal experience integrating twelve-step principles and practice with recovery from sexual child abuse.)

Small, Fred

1994 *Promises Worth Keeping: The Songs of Fred Small, Volume II.* Cambridge, MA: Yellow Moon Press. (ISBN 0-938756-45-1. Contains "I Will Stand Fast." Yellow Moon's phone number is (617) 776-2230. Their Web site is www.yellowmoon.com)

1986 *Breaking from the Line: The Songs of Fred Small.* Cambridge, MA: Yellow Moon Press. (ISBN 0-938756-13-3. Contains "Everything Possible.")

Stephens, James

1912 *The Crock of Gold.* New York: Macmillan. ("*The Crock of Gold* is like sunlight, ozone, and high spirits. There is no book in the world in the least like it, and probably there will never be another." — *The Atlantic Monthly.* This amazing book is available as a Collier Paperback.)

Stoltenberg, John

1993 *The End of Manhood: A Book for Men of Conscience.* New York: Dutton. ("Bingo! He hits it right on the head!" — Richard, 45, Massachusetts)

Taylor, Cathryn L.

1991 *The Inner Child Workbook: What to Do with Your Past When It Just Won't Go Away.* New York: Jeremy P. Tarcher.

Terkel, Studs

1992 *Race: How Blacks and Whites Think and Feel about the American Obsession.* New York: New Press.

Tilleraas, Perry

1988 *The Color of Light: Meditations for All of Us Living with AIDS.* San Francisco: Harper & Row.

Vachss, Andrew

1993 *Another Chance to Get It Right: A Children's Book for Adults.* Milwaukie, OR: Dark Horse Publishing. (This book may be the easiest introduction to the extraordinary, but often painful, work of Andrew Vachss. I hesitated to include his works in the resource list — especially his crime novels — because they are so dark and contain so much violence and suffering. But they are so very well written. Vachss "gets it" about the damage of abuse, about blame and responsibility, and he doesn't mince words. Burke, his protagonist, is himself a survivor. Strong, courageous, and angry through his pain, he calls things as he sees them and takes whatever action is necessary. All the books in this series focus on some aspect of child abuse. I advise you not to read them when you're feeling shaky or isolated.)

W., Bill

1996 *A Simple Program: A Contemporary Translation of the Original Big Book of Alcoholics Anonymous.* New York: Hyperion. (The bible of twelve-step recovery.)

W., Nancy

1992 *Embracing the Journey: Affirmations for Living Life as a Sexual Abuse Survivor.* San Francisco: HarperCollins.

Wiehe, Vernon R.

1990 *Sibling Abuse: Hidden Physical, Emotional, and Sexual Trauma.* Lexington, MA: Lexington Books.

Williams, Strephon Kaplan

1985 *The Dreamworks Manual: A Step by Step Introduction to Working with Dreams.* Berkeley, CA: Journey Press.

Wood, Douglas

1993 *Paddle Whispers.* Duluth, MN: Pfeifer-Hamilton. ("This book is a series of essays written while the author was on a solo canoe trip in the Boundary Waters Canoe Area Wilderness in northern Minnesota." — Erik, 47, South Dakota)

The Healing Woman. A monthly publication by Healing Woman, Moss Beach, CA.

Also cited are:

Renee Fredrickson's recovery series audiotapes and her video-tape on Post Traumatic Stress Syndrome, and various tapes from twelve-step programs.

The song "I Will Stand Fast" is on Fred Small's album of the same name on the Flying Fish label (#70491). Fred's recordings are available in record stores and by mail order from Small Potatoes, P.O. Box 0765, Acton, MA 01720-0765. Phone: (508) 263-6072.

The music of Nancy Day, including her album *Survivor*, is available in some record stores and by mail order from Nancy Day, P.O. Box 1818, Haverhill, MA 01831.

Bill McKinley's beautiful album, *Everything Possible*, is available from Everything Possible, P.O. Box 1483, Indianapolis, IN 46206-1483. Phone: (317) 631-6703.

The albums of The Flirtations are widely available in good record stores, or from P.O. Box 655, Provincetown, MA 02657. E-mail: flirts@mail1.wn.net

The extraordinary musical *Into the Woods* by Stephen Sondheim and James Lapine is available on video. You will be amazed by this brilliant interpretation of abuse, recovery, and redemption told through familiar fairy tales. The original cast recording, with libretto, is available from RCA Victor.

Mariah Carey's song "Hero" is on her album *Music Box*, released by Columbia.

> **"One of the best resources I've found is the National Library of Medicine in Washington, D.C. Their computer search files have enormous amounts of data on sexual child abuse and PTSD!" — Jim, 42, New Hampshire**

OTHER RESOURCES

So as not to duplicate the resource list in *Victims No Longer*, most of the organizations and newsletters were included in this section because:

1. they were suggested by male survivors, or

2. their staff members wrote to me asking to be included, or

3. they have come into being (or undergone significant changes) since the publication of the other book.

Although far more extensive than the one in *Victims No Longer*, this list is far from exhaustive — new resources are developing and old ones are changing all the time. Some of these organizations may no longer be operating by the time you read this. I tried to provide accurate up-to-date listings at the time of publication, concentrating on nonprofit organizations. **Please understand that inclusion in this list does not constitute my endorsement of any person, program, or service.** Wherever possible, I used the descriptive language that was sent to me, or excerpted it from their literature. Note that some local chapters or meetings of an organization may be better than others. If you are interested in any of these resources, please investigate them carefully, and trust your own best judgment about what is right for you.

If other institutions, programs, groups, or services have aided your recovery, please let me know, so I can add them to my referral list.

WORLD WIDE WEB SITES

The Internet can be an important resource for male survivors, especially those who are geographically isolated or who are not yet able to be open and visible about the abuse they experienced in childhood. While there is a good deal of valuable information and support available on the Internet, there is also fraud, misrepresentation, and danger. Individuals and organizations may not be as they represent themselves. Please take your time, use caution and your own best judgment.

Higher Education Center against Violence and Abuse

http://www.umn.edu/~mincava/ca.html

Clearinghouse featuring fact sheets, information resources, and other links.

The Invisible Boy: Revisioning the Victimization of Male Children and Teens

http://www.travel-net.com/~pater/invis.htm

This is an on-line book prepared by Frederick Matthew, Ph.D., Community Psychologist at Central Toronto Youth Services for The National Clearinghouse on Family Violence, Health Canada, March 1996. Its sections include: Introduction: Opening the Door to Male Victims; Prevalence: A Many-Sided Story; Perpetrators of Male Victimization; Effects of Victimization on Males; Implications; Resources and Bibliography.

It's my party and I'll cry if I want to

http://users.netaccess.co.nz/amv/abuse/abuse.htm

Andrew Moffatt-Vallance, a male survivor in New Zealand, created this highly personal, powerful, and interesting Web site that focuses on abuse by female offenders. He introduces the site with the following disclaimer: "This site is not endorsed by anyone other than myself. The opinions expressed here are entirely my own. The subject matter here deals with child sexual abuse by female offenders and by its very nature may in part be graphic and explicit. While this site is specifically intended to 'speak to' the survivors of female abusers, everyone is most welcome here. If you've been abused, you're a survivor, and I welcome you and hope you might find something useful here (even if it's just a link)."

Male Abuse Survivors Support Forum (MASSF)

www.noahgrey.com/massf

"The Male Abuse Survivors Support Forum (MASSF) is an on-line safe haven and ever growing community of support for male survivors of sexual and physical abuse. Includes an extensive collection of survivor stories, a gallery of survivors' poetry and artwork, and more.... MASSF is primarily a discussion and fellowship area for male survivors of abuse. I would like to emphasize, though, that the site is open to *everyone* with an interest in and concern for the subject... The MASSF is not a charity, nor is it affiliated with any organization.... Please feel free to speak your mind here (you may post as 'Anonymous' if you wish, and you need not give any information about yourself you're uncomfortable giving); this forum is here for *you*, whether you want to tell your story or just share something in your heart.... Above and beyond all else, we want this to be a place where you may feel safe, and free at all times to share whatever is in your heart — all of us have 'been there,' all of us know the feelings...and all of us are here for each other." —Noah Grey

Four Web sites for survivors and allies, added just before printing to replace a site that no longer exists:
The Child Trauma Academy (formerly Civitas)
    http://www.childtrauma.org
The Healing Woman
    http://www.healing woman.org
Sidran Foundation
    http://www.sidran.org
The Zero (Official Homepage of Andrew Vachss)
    http://www.vachss.com/

Sexual Abuse of Males: Prevalence, Lasting Effects, and Resources
    http://www.jimhopper.com/male-ab
Jim Hopper is a psychologist with extensive experience in therapy and research with male and female survivors of sexual child abuse. He is also an Internet wizard and a good person. Dr. Hopper has created an excellent Web site for survivors, professionals, and other allies. Check out this site. In Jim Hopper's own words:
"My main philosophy is about empowering men to educate themselves, particularly letting them know about work professionals and researchers have been doing to try to understand and help others like themselves. Here are the reasons I have published this page:
"1. To help those looking for Web resources on the sexual abuse of boys and the lasting effects of childhood sexual abuse in the lives of men.
"2. To inform men who were sexually abused in childhood and want to know what professional researchers and therapists have learned, but who might not otherwise seek information in scholarly journals and books.
"3. To help people understand how researchers come up with statistics on child sexual abuse, because the popular media foster confusion and most people don't read scholarly journals where researchers publish their work."

Sexual Assault Information Page

http://www.cs.utk.edu/~bartley/saInfoPage.html

Links to national organizations and resources for acquaintance rape, sexual child abuse, crime victim compensation, domestic violence, posttraumatic stress disorder, and sexual assault centers. Publishes an E-mail newsletter.

Social Work Access Network (SWAN)

http://www.sc.edu/swan/

Links to resources about adoption, AIDS/HIV, substance abuse, child abuse and neglect, domestic violence, mental health, and youth violence.

The Wounded Healer

http://idealist.com/wounded_healer/

Links for psychotherapists and others who are survivors of child abuse and other trauma.

Other Web sites have been included as part of the organizational listings that follow.

ORGANIZATIONS LISTED APLHABETICALLY BY COUNTRIES

ARGENTINA:

Fundacion Precavida (Branch of Self-Help Clearinghouse)
Espinosa 1885, 2nd Floor, "B" Capital Federal, Buenos Aires
Phone: (01) 582-8680; Fax: (01) 951-5925
Coordinators: Luis Kuncenicz and Dora Kapeluschnik

AUSTRALIA:

Advocates for Survivors of Child Abuse (ASCA)
P. O. Box 842, Darlinghurst, New South Wales 2010
Phone: (02) 9360-7281 or (02) 1800-657-380; Fax: (02) 9331-2487
E-mail: watson@fastlink.com.au
Web site: www.fastlink.com.au/clients/asca/ASCA.html
"...an Australian national organisation, for men and women, dedicated to serving the needs of adult survivors of child abuse...ASCA's goal is to break the silence, so that healing becomes available for all and so end the cycle of abuse for the benefit of the next generation."

Provides: Advocacy, education, support meetings for survivors and friends, and monthly newsletter.

Brisbane Rape & Incest Crisis Centre
14 Brook Street, Highgate Hill, Brisbane, Queensland 4101
Phone: (07) 3846-1206

Canberra Rape Crisis Centre
P.O. Box 916, Dickson, Australian Capital Territory 2602
Phone: (06) 247-2525

Collective of Self-Help Groups
P. O. Box 251, Brunswick East, Victoria 3057
Phone: (03) 388-1777

Eastern and Central Sexual Assault Services
Level 5, Building 72, Royal Prince Alfred Hospital, Missendon Road, Camperdown, New South Wales 2050
Phone: (02) 9515-7566; Fax: (02) 9515-8106
Provides: Individual counselling and groups for male survivors, information, and referrals.
Contact: Tony Phiskie

Incest and Ritual Abuse Library
114 South Street, Freemantle, Western Australia 6160
Phone: (08) 8825-3550
Open Fridays 1pm–4pm.

Men Embracing Nonviolent Solutions (MENS)
Berwickwide Community Health Service, 67 Power Road, Doveton, Victoria 3177
Phone: (03) 9791-5700 or (03) 9700-4501; Men's Referral Service: (03) 9428-2899.
Provides: Programs for men, including support groups, structured programs on anger and violence, Speak Out And Recover (SOAR) a recovery group for adult male survivors of childhood sexual abuse, alcohol and drug counselling, problem gambling counselling, referrals and speakers to community groups and institutions. "All calls are treated confidentially."
Contact: Rod Shearer

Mens Counselling Service
P.O. Box 1031, Fitzroy North, Victoria 3068
Phone: (03) 9489-1010
   Provides: Counselling, groups for male survivors, information, referrals, public education, workshops, and professional trainings.
Contact: Chris Dawson

Northern Centre Against Sexual Assault
Austin & Repatriation Medical Centre
Austin Campus, Studley Road, Heidelberg, Victoria
Phone: (03) 9459-3190
E-mail: ncasa@austin.unimelb.edu.au
Web site: http://www.northern.casa.org.au
   Provides: Individual and family counselling, time limited groups for adult male survivors and adolescents, training for professionals, information, and referrals.

Nth Sexual Assault Group
P.O. Box 1062, Lauceston, Tasmania 7250

Rainbow Male Survivors Network (RMSN)
P.O. Box 2186, Richmond South, Victoria, 3121
E-mail: rainbownet@yarranet.net.au
Web site: http://yarranet.net.au/rmsn/rainbownet.htm
   "...a survivor initiated and administered network organisation for gay and bisexual males who have survived sexual abuse."
   Provides: Referral service throughout Victoria, facilitated support group for gay and bisexual male survivors, information concerning sexual abuse of gay and bisexual men for support agencies, newsletter, and advocacy services for male survivors.

Sexual Assault Referral Centre
Shop 25, Ground Floor, Casuarina Plaza, Casuarina, Darwin, Northern Territory 0810

Sexual Assault Resource Centre
Perth, Western Australia
Phone: (08) 9340-1828; (1-800) 199-888

Sexual Assault Support Service
P.O. Box 217, North Hobart, Tasmania 7002
Contact: Jo Flanagan

Support Network for Men
P.O. Box 2186, Richmond South, Victoria 3121
Phone: (03) 9437-9736
Contact: Allan

#Survivors on the Net Australia, Inc.
E-mail: info@survivors.org.au
Web site: www.survivors.org.au
"We collect petitions at shopping malls to shape change to local laws. (Since August 12, 1997) I have met probably in excess of two thousand male survivors and half of those would be disclosing for the first time. Also in that time I would have met about four thousand female survivors, half of those would also be disclosing for the first time. The youngest of either gender was eleven, the eldest eighty-seven. It has been a privilege to be so trusted."

Western Institute of Self-Help
80 Railway Street, Cottesloe, Western Australia 6011
Phone: (09) 383-3188; Fax: 09-385-1476
Branch of Self-Help Clearinghouse
Director: Denise Kelly

Yarrow Place Rape and Sexual Assault Service
P.O. Box 620, North Adelaide, South Australia 5066
Phone: (08) 8226-8777

AUSTRIA:

Servicestelle für Selbsthilfegruppen
Schottenring 24, Vienna, A-1160
Phone: (01) 81223; Fax (01) 998-1221
Director: Ilse Forster

BELGIUM:

Trefpunt Zelf Hulp
E. Van Evenstraat 2 C, Leuven, 3000
Phone: (016) 23-65-07; Fax: (016) 32-33-65
Director: Linda Verwimp

CANADA:

Anonymous Sexual Abuse Recovery [Canada] (ASAR[C])
Phone: (905) 765-5769 (9am–5pm)
E-mail: donwin@asar.org
Web site: http://www.worldchat.com/public/asarc/
"...a free on-line service facilitating self-help support to victims and survivors of the trauma of sexual abuse and/or sexual assault."

Provides: BBS (Bulletin Board Service), including Open Forum, Survivors' Support Forum, Professionals Forum and Friends' Forum; On-line Library, local referral service for Southern Ontario and links to external Web sites.

East Prince Child Sexual Abuse Coalition
P.O. Box 1648, Summerside, Prince Edward Island C1N 2V5
Phone: (902) 436-9171; Fax: 902-888-8247

A coalition of professionals committed to issues of support, public education, treatment, and recovery in the area of child sexual abuse — including male survivor issues.

Provides: Information, referrals and occasional workshops on topics that have included institutional abuse and male survivor issues.

Family Life Education Council
233 12th Avenue, S.W., Calgary, Alberta T2R 0G9
Phone: (403) 262-1117; Fax: 403-261-2813

A branch of the Self-Help Clearinghouse.

Prince Edward Island Self-Help Clearinghouse
Box 785, Charlottetown, Prince Edward Island C1A 7L9
Phone: (902) 566-3034; Fax: (902) 566-4643
E-mail: faulk@cycor.ca

Self-Help Connection
Mental Health Association, 63 King Street, Dartmouth, Nova Scotia B2Y 2R7
Phone: (902) 466-2011; Fax: (902) 466-3300

Self-Help Resource Centre
40 Orchard View Blvd. — Suite 219, Toronto, Ontario M4R 1B9
Phone: (416) 487-4355; Fax: (416) 487-0624

Serves Greater Toronto area. Lists other Ontario clearinghouses.

Sexually Abused Males Surviving (S.A.M.S.)
47 Campbell Road, Kentville, Nova Scotia B4N 1Y1
Phone: (902) 678-2913
"SAMS is a self-help support group for men who have suffered childhood sexual abuse, or any other type of sexual abuse. Founded by survivors for survivors."
Contact: Jerry

Sexual Assault Recovery Anonymous (SARA)
P.O. Box 16, Surrey, British Columbia V3T 4W4

Vancouver Society for Male Survivors of Sexual Abuse
311-1008 Homer Street, Vancouver, BC V6B 2X1
Phone: (604) 682-6482
"...a nonprofit society, established to provide therapeutic services for males who have been sexually abused at some time in their lives."
Provides: Treatment, support services, educational materials, and consultation.

Vis-à-Vis
Canadian Council on Social Development
441 MacLaren, 4th Floor, Ottawa, Ontario K2P 2H3
Phone: (613) 236-8977
Provides: National family violence newsletter.

Winnipeg Self-Help Resource Clearinghouse
NorWest Coop & Health Centre
103-61 Tyndall Avenue, Winnipeg, Manitoba R2X 2T4
Phone: (204) 589-5500 or (204) 633-5955

CROATIA:

College of Nursing (Branch of Self-Help Clearinghouse)
University of Zagreb, Mlinarska 38, Zagreb, Y-41000
Phone: (041) 28-666
Contact: Arpad Barath

DENMARK: (These listings are all connected to the Self-Help Clearinghouse.)

Center for Frivilligt Socialt Arbejde
Pantheonsgade 5.3, Odense C, 5000
Phone: (066) 14-60-61; Fax: (066) 14-20-17
Executive Director: Ulla Habermann, National Volunteer Centre

Lailos — National
Tordenjkjoldsvei 20, Helsinor, 3000
Coordinator: Ulla-Britta Buch

Selvhjaelps-Grupper Centre in Kolding
Vesterskovog 19, Bjest, 6091
Director: Lisbeth Bonde Petersen

Social Radgivning og Bistand
Sortedam Dosseringen 3, st. th., Kobenhavn N, 2200
Phone: 31-31-71-97
Director: Birthe Gamst; Coordinator: Ann Gamst

ENGLAND: (See separate listings for Northern Ireland, Scotland, and Wales.) Many thanks to Alastair Hilton of First Step, Leicester, who researched much of the information for Great Britain. He also suggested the following: "If you cannot find any help in your area, you could try contacting your local Social Services Department or Citizens Advice Bureau. They should have up-to-date information of any new services in your area. New projects for male survivors are starting on an increasing scale so don't give up just yet. Failing that, try one of the other organisations listed below. They may be able to help."

Accuracy About Abuse:
P.O. Box 3125, London, NW3 5QB
Phone: (0171) 431-5339; Fax: (0171) 431-3101
E-mail: orr@aaastar.demon.co.uk
    Provides: Newsletter, research, information, and networking support for survivors, professionals, and activists working in the field of child abuse, incest, and ritual abuse. "Aims to get an accurate picture of abuse across to the public."
Contact: Marjorie Orr

Andover Rape Crisis Helpline (ARCH)
Phone: (01264) 336-222

Provides: "Counselling for women and men who have been raped or sexually abused." Serves Hampshire. Hours: Tuesday 7pm–9pm; Saturday 2pm-4pm.

Avon Sexual Abuse Centre
P.O. Box 665, Bristol, BS99 1XY
Phone: (0117) 935-1707
"Free and confidential short-term counselling for young and adult women and men who have been sexually abused...Groups are also sometimes available."

Basingstoke Rape and Sexual Abuse Crisis Centre
Phone: (01256) 840-224; Textphone: (01256) 814-555
"Serves Hampshire and West Surrey. Provides helpline for anyone (over fifteen) who has been sexually abused or assaulted, including partners and families."
Provides: Information, advice, counselling, referrals and listening. Face-to-face counselling and support available. Hours: Tuesday-Thursday 7pm–10pm.

Campaign for the Rights Of Sexual abuse Survivors (C.R.O.S.S.)
c/o 29a Rye Hill Park, Peckham, London SE15
Phone: (0181) 452-6504
Hours: Monday, Tuesday, Thursday, Friday 6pm–9pm.
Please enclose an S.A.S.E.

Child Helpline
Phone: (0800) 919-300 (Freephone)
Provides: Advice, listening support and counselling for young people who have been/are being sexually abused. Serves South Yorkshire, Derbyshire, and surrounding areas. Hours: Monday–Friday 7pm–10pm.

Childhood Abuse Advisory Service (CAAS)
Phone: (01255) 435-000 (Essex); (01376) 519-800 (North London)
Provides: Advice, information and listening for adult (16+) survivors of childhood sexual abuse. Serves Essex and North London. Hours: Monday–Friday 9am–6pm.

Childwatch
206 Hessle Road, Hull, HU3 3BE
Phone: (01482) 32552 or (01482) 216681
   Provides: Telephone counselling for adults who have been abused as children and their families. Monday–Wednesday 10am–3pm; Tuesday 7pm–10pm.

Choices (Cambridge)
Phone: (01223) 467-897
   "Listening service for women who were sexually abused in childhood." At the time this was written they were developing a service for men. Serves Cambridgeshire and parts of Suffolk. Hours: Tuesday 12:30pm–2:30pm; Thursday 6pm–8pm.

Chorley and South Ribble Rape and Sexual Abuse Helpline (CRASH)
Phone: (01257) 267-776
   Provides: Information, support, and advice for people who have been raped/sexually assaulted. Serves Chorley, South Ribble, and surrounding districts. Hours: Tuesday 7pm–9:30pm.

Cornwall Rape and Sexual Abuse Centre
Phone: (01872) 265-2100
   Provides: Advice and support for men, women and children (13+) who have been raped/sexually abused. Serves Cornwall and the Isles of Scilly. Hours: Monday, Tuesday, Thursday, Friday 9:30am–11:30am; Monday, Wednesday 7pm–10pm.

Counselling and Recovery Line
Phone: (0151) 420-0494
   "Counselling, advice, and information for men on all issues, particularly sexual abuse and rape." Serves Halton area. Hours: 24 hours everyday.

Derby Rape Crisis
Phone: (01332) 372-545
   Provides: Information and support for adults who have been raped or sexually abused. Serves Derbyshire. Hours: Monday 10am–12noon; Thursday 7:30pm–9:30pm; Friday 1pm–3pm.

Directory and Book Services (DABS)
79 Copley Road, Doncaster, South Yorkshire, DN1 2QP
Phone and Fax: (01302) 768-689
Provides: "...a fast and confidential mail-order service, specialising in books on survivor issues. They also produce a Survivors Pack. (Includes current book list, helpsheet, and a list of your local organisations). Free on request.
DABS National Resource Directory [is] an up-to-date directory of over 300 organisations in England, Scotland, and Wales: rape crisis centres, telephone helplines, social service departments, self-help groups, etc. DABS also gives free advice about local services.

Doncaster Rape and Sexual Abuse Counselling Centre
Phone: (01302) 360-421
Provides: Counselling and information for male and female survivors of sexual violence. Serves Doncaster and surrounding areas. Hours: Monday 1pm–4pm; Wednesday 6pm–8pm.

EMERGE
Phone: (01785) 225-991; (01543) 576-174
Provides: Support for adult survivors of childhood sexual abuse. Serves Staffordshire. Hours: Monday–Friday 7pm–10pm.

Family Matters
5 Manor Road, Gravesend, Kent, DA12 1AA
Phone: (01474) 537-392
Provides: Helpline for anyone who has experienced sexual abuse in childhood. Offers counselling, listening, and information to adults and children aged eight and over. Available daily 10am–12 noon, 2pm–4pm, 7pm–8:30pm.

First Step
Leicester FSU, 26 Severn Street, Leicester, LE2 0NN
Phone: (0116) 254-3352; Fax: (0116) 275-5216
Helpline: (0116) 255-8868 (available Monday 7–10 pm. Answerphone at other times. All calls returned.)
"Help for adult male survivors of childhood sexual abuse or male rape, and their supporters."
Newsletter: "...welcomes contributions from those who have something to share with male survivors, their supporters, and professionals."

Provides: Telephone helpline, face-to-face and group support for survivors, families, partners, and carers living in the City of Leicester, Leicestershire, and Rutland. Will respond to telephone calls from other areas. Consultation and training for service providers, newsletter, book reviews, and "developing an individual and group work service for sexually abused boys up to the age of eighteen. Referrals of young male survivors are welcome."

Contact: John Roberts or Alastair Hilton

Grimsby Rape Crisis
Phone: (01472) 322-111

Provides: Counselling, advice and support for women and men who have been raped, sexually abused, or assaulted. Serves Lincolnshire area, including Scunthorpe, Grimsby, Cleethorpes. Hours: Wednesday 7pm–9pm.

Incest and Sexual Abuse Survivors Group (ISAS)
Phone: (01636) 610-313

"Serves the area of North Nottinghamshire. Helpline available Monday–Friday 7pm–9:30pm. For survivors of incest and sexual abuse (18+), their relatives and partners."

Provides: counselling, listening, information, and advice. Face-to-face counselling available.

Justice for Abused Children
Phone: (0191) 221-1919

Provides: Listening for adult survivors of childhood abuse, their partners and parents. Serves Tyne and Wear, Durham. Hours: Monday–Friday 11am–2pm.

Luton and District Rape Crisis Centre
Phone: (01582) 733-592

"Available Monday–Friday 10am–4pm. Answerphone at other times. Returns all calls."

Provides: Telephone counselling, information, advice, and referrals for anyone over fifteen who has been raped or sexually abused. Face-to-face counselling also available. Serves Bedfordshire and parts of Hertfordshire.

Male Survivors Oxford
Phone: (01491) 833-474
"Serves Thames Valley area. Telephone helpline and face-to-face counselling available. Answerphone messages checked hourly."

MASH (Men As Survivors Helpline)
c/o Vicky Abel, Victim Support, 36 Dean Lane, Bedminster, Bristol BS3
Phone: (0117) 907-7100
"Telephone counselling for male survivors of childhood and adult sexual abuse and rape. Male and female counsellors are available. Helpline open Thursday 7pm–9 pm." Serves Bristol and South West England.

NAPSAC
Department of Learning Disabilities, Floor E, South Block, University Hospital, Nottingham, NG7 2UH
Phone: (0115) 970-9987
Provides: "Information and advice on all aspects of the sexual abuse/exploitation of adults and children with learning difficulties, for parents and involved professionals...produces a wide range of publications." Monday–Friday 8:30am–4:30pm.

National Child Protection Helpline (NSPCC)
42 Curtain Road, London, EC2A 3NH
Phone: (0800) 800-500 (Freephone); (0800) 056-0566 (Textphone)
Helpline offers counselling, information, and advice. Serves England, Wales, and Northern Ireland. 24 hours every day.

Portsmouth Area Rape Crisis Service
P.O. Box 3, Portsmouth, Hants. P01
Phone: (01705) 669-516 (Men's Line)
"Serves Portsmouth and S.E. Hampshire area."
Provides: Helpline, advice, information, referrals, and face-to-face counselling. Also arranges support groups. Available Wednesday and Friday. 7pm–10pm. Answerphone at other times.
Contact: Darrell Gale

Rape and Sexual Abuse Support Centre (Guildford)
Phone: (01483) 810-099

Provides: Support, counselling, information, advice for men and women who have been raped or sexually abused. Serves Surrey, parts of Hampshire, and West Sussex. Hours: Monday, Wednesday, Thursday, Sunday 7pm–10pm.

Rape and Sexual Violence Project
Phone: (0121) 643-5600

Provides: Counselling, advice, and information for women and men who have been raped or sexually abused. Serves Birmingham. Hours: Monday–Thursday 10am–10pm; Friday 10am–2pm.

Rape, Examination, Advice, Counselling, Help (REACH)
Phone: (0191) 226-0825; Textphone: (0191) 272-0844

Provides: Support for women (16+) and men who have been raped or recently sexually assaulted. Serves Northumberland, Tyne, and Wear. Variable opening times.

Respond
24-32 Stephenson Way, 3rd Floor, London, NW1 2HD
Phone: (0171) 383-0700

Provides: "Telephone service for carers and professionals who are supporting people with learning disabilities who have been sexually abused. Offers consultancy and referrals to psychotherapy and risk assessment services. Also provides support for people with learning disabilities who have experienced or perpetrated sexual abuse." Hours: Monday–Friday 9am–5pm.

SAFE
P.O. Box 1557, Salisbury, SP1 2TP
Phone: (01722) 410-889

"Helpline for people who have been abused in a ritual setting. Offers support and information." Hours: Monday, Wednesday, Thursday 9:30am–11:30am; Tuesday, Wednesday, Friday 7:30pm–9:30pm; Saturday 3:30pm–5:30pm.

Sage Positive
Phone: (0149)1 839-538

"Wallingford (Serves Thames Valley Area)."

Provides: A range of individual and group therapies for survivors, families, and partners.

Sanctuary
Phone: (01634) 378-300
Provides: Counselling for anyone affected by sexual abuse. Serves Kent and Essex. Hours: Monday–Saturday 9am–10pm.

SAVS
Phone: (01204) 364-683
Provides: Information and listening for adults who have experienced childhood sexual abuse. Serves Greater Manchester area. Hours: Monday–Friday 9am–9pm.

Scunthorpe Rape Crisis
Phone: (01724) 853-953
Provides: Counselling, advice, and support for women and men who have been raped, sexually abused, or assaulted. Serves Lincolnshire. Hours: Monday 7pm–9pm; Thursday 8pm–10pm.

Self-Help Team
20 Pelham Road, Nottingham, NG5 1AP
Phone: (0115) 969-1212; Fax: (0115) 960-2049
Team Leader: Judy Wilson

Sexual Abuse and Incest Victims Emerge (SAIVE)
Phone: (01782) 265-839
"Serves Stoke on Trent and surrounding areas. Information, advice, and a listening service for anyone who has experienced sexual abuse. Includes partners and families. Also offers face-to-face counselling if required. Available 10am–5pm Monday–Friday. Answerphone redirects callers and allows messages to be left."

South Cumbria Rape and Abuse Service
Phone: (01539) 734-743
Provides: Information and listening. Staffed by women (Mondays 7pm–9pm) and men (one Wednesday per month 7pm–8:30pm). Serves South Cumbria and Furness.

Survive

Rooms 9/10, Floor 2, Breeden House, Edleston Road, Crewe, CW2 7EA

Phone: (01270) 253-179 (Monday, Wednesday); (01606) 79796 (Thursday)

"Helpline for male and female survivors (14+) of sexual abuse. Offers information, advice, and referrals to local counsellors." Serves North West England. Hours: Monday and Thursday 1pm–4pm; Wednesday 6:30pm–9pm.

Survivors (Bedfordshire, Luton)

Phone: (01582) 410-688

"Helpline for men: Thursday 7pm–10pm. Individual and group support available. There's a survivor group when there are enough men who want one."

Survivors (London)

For Male Victims of Sexual Abuse

P.O. Box 2470, London W2 1NW

Phone: (0181) 340-6118 (office); (0171) 833-3737 (helpline)

"...a self-help organisation...national support organisation working with any male victim or survivor of sexual violence..." A Registered Charity.

Provides: Telephone helpline Tuesday and Wednesday 7pm–10pm, facilitated male survivor groups, free face-to-face counselling, public, professional, and media education, especially on issues of male rape.

Survivors (Sheffield)

P.O. Box 142, Sheffield, S1 3HG

Phone: (0114) 279-6333

"Counselling service for sexually abused men and male partners of victims of abuse or rape. If you need to talk to someone, our counsellors are here to listen and believe. You will not be judged, condemned, or told what to do. We offer a safe and supportive environment. The service is confidential and free."

Provides: Free telephone and face-to-face counselling for male survivors of sexual abuse and rape, support groups, very useful Self-Help Pack, counselling for partners, trainings for volunteers and professional organisations. Serves South Yorkshire. Hours: Monday 6pm–8pm.

Survivors (Swindon)
c/o Focus, 25 Morley Street, Swindon, SN1 1SG
Phone: (01793) 878-316
　　Provides: Support group, individual counselling and "helpline for adult (17+) male survivors of child sex abuse and adult rape. Offers advice, information, and listening support. Answerphone messages are returned as soon as possible." Provides training to other organisations. Serves South East and South West England. Hours: Wednesday 7pm–9pm.

Survivors' Coalition
52-54 Featherstone Street, London, EC1 8RT
　　"A coalition of female and male survivors and survivors' groups who are campaigning together to: change the legal system to protect the rights of survivors; lobby for resources for healing; counter misinformation in the media; educate professionals to ensure more effective care for survivors."
Provides: Newsletter "Fighting Back" and resource lists for Great Britain and Ireland.

Survivors Directory
Broadcasting Support Services,
Westminster House, 11 Portland Street, Manchester, M1 3HU
Phone: (016)1 455-1212; Fax: (0161) 455-0066
　　"A national resource offering detailed information of groups working on issues of sexual violence. Contains hundreds of contact addresses and phone numbers."
　　Provides: A directory listing organisations in Great Britain and Ireland.

#Survivors on the Net
321 Portland Road, Hove, East Sussex, BN3 5SE
Phone: (01273) 410-622
E-mail: info@survivors.org.uk
Web site: http://www.survivors.org.uk/
　　"Provide support and information on the Internet for survivors of childhood abuse, their partners, family and friends by: providing an up-to-date and comprehensive database of self-help groups, freephone numbers, counsellors, and therapists; establishing a twenty-four hour information and self-help forum for survivors run by

survivors; providing a Web site with links to other resources available both locally and on the Internet; establish an E-mail enquiry and support service; monthly newsletter on the Web site free to download as hard copy."

Survivors Support
c/o South Side Family Project, 36 St. Michaels Road, Whiteway, Bath BA2 1PZ
Phone: (01225) 482-368 or (01225) 331-243
"One-to-one counselling for male/female survivors of sexual abuse or rape. Group work also available. Open during office hours, plus some evenings."

Telephone Helplines Directory
The Resource Information Service,
The Basement, 38 Great Pulteney Street, London W1R 3DE
Phone: (0171) 494-2408
"The only national source of information specifically about helplines in the United Kingdom. Provides details of approximately one thousand national, regional, and local helplines throughout England, Wales, Scotland, and Northern Ireland. Published by the Telephone Helplines Association."

Victim Support (Wolverhampton)
Phone: (01902) 427-223
"Available Monday–Friday 9am–5pm. Offers telephone service to anyone (18+) who has experienced rape or sexual assault. Includes information, advice and appointments for counselling. Answerphone available — all calls returned. Serves Wolverhampton and surrounding areas.

VOICE
P.O. Box 238, Derby, DE1 1HA
Phone: (01332) 519-872 (Helpline Monday–Friday 9 am–5 pm)
"A national support and information group for people with learning disabilities who have been abused, their families and carers. Also campaigns for changes in the law and practice."

Warrington Rape Crisis
Phone: (01925) 245-444

Provides: Counselling, advice, and information for women and men who have experienced sexual violence. Hours: Monday and Thursday 6:30pm–8:30pm, Wednesday 1pm–3pm.

Winchester Rape Crisis
Phone: (01962) 848-024 (Women); (01962) 848-027 (Men)
Provides: Listening and support for women and men who have been raped and/or sexually abused. Serves mainly Hampshire. Hours: Tuesday 7pm–9:30pm (women); Thursday 7pm–9:30pm (men and women).

Working With Men
320 Commercial Way, London SE15 1QN
"For professionals working with men."

FRANCE:

S.O.S. Inceste
B.P. 345, Grenoble Cedex 38013
Phone: (076) 47-90-93

GERMANY: (The following listings are of national self-help clearinghouses. Check with them for the 100+ local German clearinghouses.)

Deutsche Arsseitsgemeinschaft Selbsthilfegruppen (DAG SHG)
c/o Friedrichstraße 28, Giessen, D-6300
Phone: (0641) 702-2478
Contact: Jürgen Matzat

Nationale Kontakt und Informationsstelle zur Anregung und Unterstutzung von Selbsthilfegruppen (NAKOS)
Albrecht-Achilles-Straße 65, Berlin, D-10709
Phone: (030) 891-4019; Fax: (030) 893-4014
Director: Klaus Balke

GREECE:

Institute of Information & Research for Youth
45 Pipinou Street, Athens 112.51
Phone: (01) 821-8289; Fax: (01) 8254071
"A charity...its purpose is the prevention of drug abuse to be achieved by: a) briefing and providing information on all aspects of the problem, b) solving problems that lead to the susceptibility to drug use."

Provides: Library and information centre, research, political lobbying, overseas networking, career centre, centre on drugs, family-based intervention programme, advice to new organisations, bibliography, and social activities.

HUNGARY:

Self-Help Groups Team
National Committee of Mental Health, P. O. Box 39, Budapest, H-1525
Coordinator: Ms. Zsuzsa

IRELAND:

C.A.R.I. Foundation
2 Garryowen Road, St. Johns, Limerick, 061
Phone: (061) 413-331; (061) 00764

Dublin Rape Crisis Centre
70, Lwr Leeson Street, Dublin 2
Contact: John Brophy

ISRAEL:

National Self-Help Clearinghouse
37 King George Street, P. O. Box 23223, Tel Aviv, 61231
Phone: (03) 299389
Director: Martha Ramon

Tel Aviv Rape Crisis Centre
P.O. Box 3117, Tel Aviv 61030
Phone: (03) 234-314; 24-Hour Hotline: (03) 234-819
"The largest centre in Israel giving assistance to women, men, and teenagers from all sectors of the population (also to tourists)

who have suffered from any form of sexual abuse, or who are in contact with someone who has, and giving information and aid on any subject related to sexual abuse...we developed and conducted a first-of-its-kind training course for men volunteers and have opened a hot line for men and boys...which functions twice a week." Serves the Dan area and the entire central region.
Contact: Rachel Naveh

JAPAN:

The Osaka Self-Help Support Center
6-998-3-3-225, Nakamozu-cho, Osaka, 591
Phone: (06) 722-57-3667; Fax: (06) 722-54-6075
Director: Takehiro Sadato; Contact: Hiroyuko Matsuda

KENYA:

Amani Counselling Centre
P.O. Box 21452, Nairobi
Contact: Sister Bernice Rigney, MM

NETHERLANDS:

European Network for Backlash Research (ENBAR)
F. Glockstraat 167, 9665BJ Oude Pekela, NL
Provides: Journal and support for activists and professionals working in the field of incest, child abuse, and ritual abuse.

NEW ZEALAND:

Essentially Men
P.O. Box 48-169, Blockhouse Bay, Auckland
Phone: (09) 627-9827
Contact: Rex McCann

The Green Light Support Service
Wellington
Contact: Gary or John (04) 564-3945 or Gary (025) 667-049

Life Line
Auckland
Phone: (09) 522-2808

Male Survivors of Sexual Abuse
Room 32, Christchurch Community House, 187 Cashel Street,
P.O. Box 22-372, Christchurch 8001
Phone: (03) 377-6747

"To enhance the recovery process with peer support for men and to provide resources for clients to aid them in changing their lives. To encourage a greater public awareness of child sexual abuse issues for male survivors. To encourage the formation of support groups and production of resources for male survivors of child abuse within New Zealand. To provide affordable access to help for survivors of child sexual abuse. To empower survivors to take control of their lives and look towards a positive future."

Provides: Monthly peer support group meeting supervised by a therapist; individual meetings with one other survivor; resource information.

Man Alive
Auckland
Phone: (09) 835-0509

Oranga–Kaha Program
Hamilton
Contact: Anton Roest (07) 843-4509 or Warrick Smith (07) 829-4731

Te Puna Oranga
5th Floor, 180 Manchester Street, P.O. Box 13-468, Christchurch
Phone: (03) 365-5715
Contact: Daniel Mataki

NORTHERN IRELAND: (See also listings for England.)

Belfast Rape Crisis and Sexual Abuse Centre
2a Donegal Street, Belfast. BT1
Phone: (01232) 249-696

"Offers telephone service to anyone who has experienced sexual abuse or violence. Available 10am–12midnight, Monday to Friday; 10am–12midnight, weekends. Also for friends, families, and partners."

Provides: Advice, counselling, information on legal and medical aspects. Referrals to and liaison with other organisations if requested.

Children's Helpline and Interlink Counselling Service
121 Spencer Road, Waterside, Londonderry BT47 1AE
Phone: (0800) 212-888 (Freephone)
   Provides: Telephone advice, information and counselling for children and adult survivors of sexual abuse. Opening hours: Monday 9am–5pm; Tuesday–Friday 9am–4pm.

NORWAY:

Support Centre Against Incest
Storgt 17, Pb 8895, Youngstorget, 0028, Oslo

POLAND:

Working Group of the Self-Help Movements
Dluga 38/40, Warszawa, 00-238
Phone: (22) 314-551; Fax: (22)314-712
Coordinator: Elzbieta Bobiatynska

SCOTLAND: (See also listings for England.)

Dunfermline Area Abuse Survivors Project
Phone: 0411 283301 (Mobile Phone)
   Provides: Support for men and women survivors of sexual abuse and incest (16+). Serves Fife area. Hours: Every day 7:30pm–9:30pm.

Dunfermline Incest Survivors Project Helpline
 Phone: (01383) 622-261
   "Helpline for anyone in the Dunfermline area who is suffering/has suffered from sexual abuse and their family and friends."
   Provides: Counselling, information, advice, listening and referrals, face-to-face counselling, a befriending service, and a self-help group. Answerphone will give times to call.

Kirkcaldy Area Abuse Survivors Project (KAASP)
Phone: (01592) 646-644
   Provides: Information, support and counselling for adult survivors (16+) of childhood sexual abuse. Serves Central Fife: Kirkcaldy, Glenrothes, Levenmouth, Kennoway, and surrounding areas. Hours: Monday–Friday 9:30am–4:30pm.

Male Survivors of Sexual Abuse (MASA)
c/o R.S.S.P.C.C.
15 Annfield Place, Glasgow, G31 2XE
Phone: (0141) 550-2048; Fax: (0141) 551-8128
 Provides: Telephone helpline and occasional group sessions for male survivors of sexual abuse. Tuesday and Friday 7pm–10 pm. Goals include "groups throughout the community, education, prevention, and training."
Contact: Bill Elliot, BA, DIP, PSW, CQSW

Open Secret (Falkirk)
Phone: (01324) 630-100
 Provides: Listening support for women and men survivors of childhood sexual abuse. Hours: Wednesday 6pm–9pm; Thursday 9am–12noon.

Rape and Sexual Abuse Line (Dingwall)
P.O. Box 10, Dingwall, Rosshire, IV15 9HE
Phone: (01349) 541-769 (staffed by women 7pm–10 pm every day) (01349) 862-686 (staffed by men Wednesdays) Can leave a message on answerphone at other times.
 "Serves mainly the Highlands and Islands area. Helpline for anyone affected by rape or abuse."
 Provides: Confidential support and listening. Will take calls from anywhere, but face-to-face available only in that area. All calls returned.

Rape Crisis Centre (Strathclyde)
Phone: (0141) 331-1990
 Provides: Support and information relating to rape, sexual assault, sexual abuse. Answerphone gives details of opening times.

SOUTH AFRICA:

Crisis Support Centre
P.O. Box 4724, Luipaardsviei 1743, 083
Phone: 227-9555
 Provides: counselling for victims of rape and abuse.

SPAIN:

Institut Municipal de la Salut (Part of Self-Help Clearinghouse)
Pa. Lesseps, 1, Barcelona, 08023
Coordinator: Francina Roca

SWEDEN:

Distriktlakare (Lapland only, part of Self-Help Clearinghouse)
Villavagan 14, Arjeplog, S-9390
Phone: 961-11230
Contact: Bo Henricson

Foreniger SCI/Stodcentrum mot Incest
Dalagatan 7, 111 23 Stockholm

SWITZERLAND:

Le Kiosque
35, Boulevard des Trancées, Geneva, CH1206
Phone: (022) 789-15
Contact: Geneviève Piret

Selbsthilfezentrum Hinderhuus
Feldbergstraße 55, Basel, CH-4057
Phone: (061) 692-8100; Fax: (061) 692-8177
Contact: Verena Vogelsanger

Team Selbsthilfe Zurich
Wilfiedstraße 7, Zurich, CH-8032
Phone: (01) 252-3036
Contact: Midi Muheim

TRINIDAD:

Adult Survivors Network
P. O. Bag 31, Belmont Post Office, Port of Spain

TURKEY:

Society for Protecting and Rehabilitation of Children from Abuse
Tibbiye Caddesi #49, 81326 Haydarpasa, Istanbul
Phone: (216) 348-0524

UNITED STATES OF AMERICA:

Above and Beyond
P.O. Box 2672, Ann Arbor, MI 48106-2672
    "...a free newsletter that reviews publications and recordings dealing with abuse."

The Alpha Foundation
Embassy Square Suite 223
2247 Palm Beach Lakes Blvd., West Palm Beach, FL 33409
Phone: (561) 688-9233
    "A group committed to the protection of boys who are abused and healing the men they become...a not-for-profit charitable organization...established to support U.N. treaties dedicated to the protection of children from abuse... includes all forms of boyhood abuse (physical, emotional, and sexual)...by...advocacy, publications, research, clinical affairs, education, and communication."
Executive Director: John Christopher Carracher, Psy.D.

American Coalition for Abuse Awareness (ACAA)
P.O. Box 27959, Washington, DC 20038-7959
Phone: (202) 462-4688; Fax: (202) 462-4689
E-mail: acaadc@aol.com
    "...a national nonpartisan coalition founded in 1993 by adult survivors and child advocates, mental health/legal professionals, and nonoffending parents to advocate for the rights of child victims and adult survivors of sexual abuse to appropriate treatment and redress through the courts. The ACAA is working towards a broad-based alliance of individuals and organizations to promote the enactment of legislation establishing the rights of children to be free of sexual victimization and exploitation."
    Provides: Legislative activity, newsletter, informational packets, judicial education, *amicus curiae* briefs, testimony, speakers, and conferences.
President and Counsel: Sherry Quirk, Esq.

National Mental Health Consumers' Self-Help Clearinghouse
1211 Chestnut Street, Suite 1207, Philadelphia, PA 19107
Phone: (800) 553-4539; Fax: (215) 636-6312
E-mail: info@mhselfhelp.org
Web site: http://www.mhselfhelp.org/

"The Clearinghouse is committed to helping mental health consumers improve their lives through self-help and advocacy. With our publications, library materials, and personal consultations, we help people establish and develop self-help groups, organize consumer coalitions, advocate for mental health reform, and fight the stigma that society places on mental illness."

The Center for the Prevention of Sexual and Domestic Violence
936 North 34th Street, Suite 200, Seattle, WA 98103
Phone: (206) 634-1903; Fax: (206) 634-0115
E-mail: cpsdv@cpsdv.org

"...is an interreligious educational program designed to equip religious leaders in addressing violence in the family, sexual assault and abuse by clergy."

Provides: Videos, written materials, workshops, and leadership training.
Executive Director: Rev. Dr. Marie M. Fortune

Childhelp, USA
15757 N. 78th Street, Scottsdale, AZ 85260
Phone: (800) 790-2445; National Child Abuse Hotline: (800) 422-4453

Provides: Education, training, consultation, networking, advocacy, and other resources for abused children. Although their Survivors of Childhood Abuse Program (SCAP) is no longer in existence, they told me that they still provide referrals for adult survivors through the Hotline.

The Cutting Edge
P.O. Box 20819, Cleveland, OH 44120

"... a newsletter that people who self-mutilate have found helpful."

Incest Survivors Resource Network International (ISRNI)
Phone: (505) 521-4260 (2pm–4pm and 11pm–midnight Eastern Time Monday–Saturday)
Web site: http://www.zianet.com/isrni
"Educational resource network run by survivors for other survivors and for professionals who work with survivors...national and international helpline...answered in person by incest-survivors only...one of the first to specifically encourage calls from adult survivors of mother-son incest."
Provides: Information about organizations and groups that support survivors as well as publications in the field. Information on starting self-help groups.

Ina Maka Family Program
United Indians of All Tribes Foundation
1945 Yale Place East, Seattle, WA 98102
Phone: (206) 325-0070
"...providing a traditional based approach to recovery for Native American Families."
Provides: Counseling, foster care, sexual abuse counseling for primary and secondary victims, crime victims advocacy, education, talking circles, and sweat lodges.
Contact: Arlene Red Elk or Jack Spotted Eagle

The Interfaith Sexual Trauma Institute (ISTI)
Saint John's Abbey and University, Collegeville, MN 56321-2000
Phone: (320) 363-3931; Fax: (320) 363-2115
E-mail: isti@csbsju.edu
Web site: http://www.csbsju.edu:80/isti/bulletin.html
"...facilitates the building of healthy, safe, and trustworthy communities of faith."
Provides: Internet Web site, newsletter, books, audiocassettes, bibliography, and workshops.
Executive Director: Fr Roman Paur, O.S.B.

C. Henry Kempe National Center for the Prevention and Treatment of Child Abuse and Neglect
1205 Oneida Street, Denver, CO 80220
Phone: (303) 321-3963
Web site: http://kempecenter.org/

The agency's primary focus is on child abuse treatment, training, and research.

Kirkridge Conference and Retreat Center
2495 Fox Gap Road, Bangor, PA 18013
Phone: (610) 588-1793; Fax: (610) 588-8510
"...has welcomed seekers of personal and social transformation since 1942." A retreat and study center in a beautiful forested ridge top location, with a supportive, respectful staff.

Provides: Workshops and retreats on a variety of topics, many with a nondenominational spiritual focus, individual retreats, and other events. [For many years, we have held our annual male survivor recovery weekends in mid-summer at Kirkridge.]
Director: Rev. Cynthia Crowner

The Linkup
1412 W. Argyle #2, Chicago, IL 60640
Phone: (773) 334-2296; Fax: (773) 334-0274
E-mail: ilinkup@aol.com
Web site: http://www.ilinkup.org
National organization of survivors of clergy abuse.

Provides: Newsletter, (Missing Link, P.O. Box 40676, Albuquerque, NM 87196. Phone: (505) 254-4634), conference, and symposiums dealing with sexual abuse, clergy sexual abuse, alcoholism and drug abuse, and awareness and prevention for professional/corporate America, the ecumenical community, and parents and educators).
Director: Rev. Thomas H. Economus, S.T.L.

M.A.L.E. (Men Assisting, Leading & Educating)
P.O. Box 460171, Aurora, CO 80046-0171
Phone: (303) 693-9930; Fax: (303) 693-6059
E-mail: male@malesurvivor.org
Web site: http://www.malesurvivor.org/
"A nonprofit organization dedicated to healing male survivors of sexual abuse...Goals: Empower male victims...provide a public presence...provide information...link male victims and families with recovery services...educate the public...prevent male sexual abuse by providing input into national and state legislation..."

Provides: Newsletter ("Men's Issues Forum"), library, informational and educational programs, national conference, and hotline. President: Shannon Sperry

The Morris Center
P.O. Box 14038, San Francisco, CA 94114-0038
Phone: (415) 452-1939; Fax: (415)452-6253
E-mail: tmc_asca@dnai.com
Web site: www.ascasupport.org

"The Morris Center for healing from child abuse is a nonprofit, 501(c)(3) tax-exempt service organization.... Our mission is to provide adult survivors of physical, sexual, or emotional child abuse with economical and effective opportunities to recover from their child abuse and to revive their identities as thrivers."

Provides: Meetings, Adult Survivors of Child Abuse (ASCA) guided self-help recovery program, manual, art and poetry events, and workshops.

Moving Forward
P.O. Box 4426, Arlington, VA 22204
Phone: (703) 271-4024; Fax: (703) 271-4025

"...a newsjournal for survivors of sexual child abuse and those who care for them...to educate our society about the effects of sexual child abuse, and to provide information about support services for survivors, significant others, and service providers."

The Next Step Counseling and Training
Mailing Address: P.O. Box 1146, Jamaica Plain, MA 02130
Phone: (617) 277-7172
E-mail: nextstep@jamaicaplain.com
Web site: http://www.abbington.com/smallwonder/index.html

In addition to individual therapy, couple counseling, and groups for male survivors, Mike Lew, Thom Harrigan, and associates are available for consultation, survivor workshops, and professional trainings. Please call for information or to be added to the mailing list for workshop announcements.

Rape Intervention Program/Crime Victim Assessment Project
St. Luke's–Roosevelt Hospital Center
411 W. 114th Street #6D, New York, NY 10025
Phone: (212) 523-4728
"For over fifteen years, we have been providing individual and group treatment to survivors of violence. Our groups are specifically designed to reduce isolation and provide a safe, healing environment for people who have been traumatized."
Provides: Free and confidential short-term groups for survivors of violent crimes, including groups for male survivors of childhood sexual abuse.
Contact: Louise Kindley or Tony Sidoti

The Safer Society Foundation
P.O. Box 340, Brandon, VT 05733-0340
Phone: (802) 247-3132; Referral Line: (802) 247-5141
Web site: http://www.safersociety.org/
"...a nonprofit agency, is a national research, advocacy, and referral center on the prevention and treatment of sexual abuse...The Safer Society Press...publishes relevant research, studies, video- and audiotapes, and books that contribute to the development of sexual abuse treatment, sexual abuse prevention, emerging topics, and developments in the field."
Provides: Computerized program network, sex offender treatment referrals, training and consultation, resource/research library, resource lists, publications, and media advocacy. Also helpful links from its Web site.
Contact: Euan Bear

Sexual Assault Treatment Center
Sinai Samaritan Medical Center
2000 W. Kilbourn Avenue, P.O. Box 342, Milwaukee, WI 53201-0342
Phone: (414) 344-0233
Among the increasing number of sexual assault treatment centers committed to understanding and support of male survivor issues.

Provides: Counseling, referrals, information, and a midsummer training institute for professionals.

Contact: Janine Arseneau, M.S.W.

Survivor Connections, Inc.

52 Lyndon Road, Cranston, RI 02905-1121

Phone: (401) 941-2548; Fax: (401) 941-2335

E-mail: totellthetruth@hotmail.com

Web site: http://www.angelfire.com/ri/totellthetruth

A nonprofit, all-volunteer operation "for survivors of sexual assault and their supportive, nonoffender relations."

Provides: Quarterly newsletter ("The Survivor Activist"), database of information on False Memory Syndrome Foundation (FMSF) members, conferences, peer support groups, merchandise.

Contact: Frank and Sara Fitzpatrick

Survivors and Victims Empowered (SAVE)

P.O. Box 3030, Lancaster, PA 17604-3030

Phone: (717) 569-3636; Fax: (717) 581-1355

Web site: http://child.cornell.edu/SAVE/home.html

"...nonprofit organization that was created to help prevent the criminal neglect and physical, emotional and sexual abuse of children and to help survivors of these childhood traumas..."

Provides: Survivors and Victims Resource Database (SVRD), Child Protection Guide (CPG), Trauma magazine for professionals and programs for abused children.

Executive Director: Philip Sheldon, Jr.

Survivors Network of Those Abused by Priests (SNAP)

8025 South Honore, Chicago, IL 60620

Phone: (312) 483-1059

"...a U.S. and Canadian self-help organization of men and women who were sexually abused by spiritual elders, e.g., Catholic priests, nuns, brothers, ministers..."

Provides:Support through local chapters, quarterly newsletter.

Trauma Recovery & Empowerment Services

c/o The Awakening Center

3166 N. Lincoln Avenue, Suite 224, Chicago, IL 60657

Phone: (773) 929-6262

Provides: Publishes the *Chicagoland Area Sexual Abuse Resource Guide for Care Providers and Consumers*, including resources for survivors nationwide and worldwide.

Director: Victoria Polin, MA

V.O.I.C.E.S. in Action, Inc.
P.O. Box 148309, Chicago, IL 60614
Phone: (312) 327-1500 or (800) 7-VOICE-8
Web site: http://www.voices-action.org/

"Victims of Incest Can Emerge Survivors...an international organization to provide assistance to victims of incest and child sexual abuse in becoming survivors and to generate public awareness of the prevalence of incest."

Provides: Newsletter, Special Interest Groups (mail support groups), national and regional conferences, publications and audiotapes, sixty-page informational "Survival Kit," and referral network.

Executive Director: Dan Stasi

Wisconsin Coalition Against Sexual Assault (WCASA)
1400 E. Washington Avenue, Suite 148, Madison, WI 53703
Phone: (608) 257-1517

Provides: Advocacy, public education, seminars for survivors, training for professionals, and "Connections," a quarterly educational newsletter.

Director: Christina Wildlake

TWELVE-STEP PROGRAMS:

There are many peer support programs based to some degree on the model of Alcoholics Anonymous. Millions who participate in these organizations consider them an invaluable part of their recovery from some form of addiction or trauma. Many other people have decided that these programs are not what they need. It is important to remember that not all meetings/groups within a program are alike. Some may meet your needs better than others; some may be safer than others. There is no guarantee, for example, that there will not be abusers attending a meeting. And not all of these organizations have an understanding of the role of sexual child abuse in addictive behaviors, or sympathy for what is necessary for recovery from the effects of sexual abuse.

If you think that a twelve-step program might be useful to you, it is a good idea to attend several different meetings at a number of locations. Once again, I urge you to follow your own judgment, accepting what makes sense to you and rejecting the rest. As I often say to survivors, nothing in recovery is mandatory except taking the best possible care of yourself. The twelve-step organizations included in the following list are all based in the United States. This list is not exhaustive, and you may be able to get more local information from your telephone directory or on the Internet. This is also true of resources outside the United States.

The following descriptions of organizations are taken from their literature. I cannot guarantee their accuracy or whether the information is up-to-date:

Survivors of Incest Anonymous (SIA)
P.O. Box 21817, Baltimore, MD 21222-6817
Phone: (410) 282-3400

"...a self-help group of men and women, eighteen years or older, who have been victims of child sexual abuse. SIA, a nonprofit organization with no dues or fees and founded in 1982, works to help victims realize that they are not responsible for what happened, and they are not alone. Members use a set of twelve suggested steps. Meetings are confidential. Members are encouraged to seek professional therapy." SIA has groups in many countries.

Incest Survivors Anonymous (ISA)
P.O. Box 17245, Long Beach, CA 90807-7245

"...an international self-help, mutual-help recovery program for men, women, and teens...run for and by survivors and their personal prosurvivors. No perpetrators or satanist individuals permitted. No professionals as professionals—only as survivors. No students as students—only as survivors...For ISA meeting, information and literature, write...stat[ing] if you are a survivor or other status...include a self-addressed stamped envelope."

Alcoholics Anonymous (AA)
475 Riverside Drive, New York, NY 10115
Phone: (212) 870-3400; TDD: (212) 870-3199; Fax: (212) 870-3003

"...an international fellowship of men and women who share their experiences with each other, so that they may solve their common

problem and help others to recover from alcoholism. The only requirement is a desire to stop drinking. There are no dues or fees for AA membership; the organization is self-supporting through member contributions. AA is not allied with any sect, denomination, politics, organization,
or institution; does not want to engage in any controversy, and neither
endorses nor opposes any causes. The primary purpose of members is
to stay sober and help other alcoholics to achieve sobriety. AA was
founded in 1935 and currently has over two million members."

Al-Anon Family Group Headquarters (Al-Anon)
Public Information Coordinator
1372 Broadway, New York, NY 10018-0862
Phone: (212) 302-7240; For free literature and information: (800)
356-9996

"Al-Anon was an adjunct of Alcoholics Anonymous until 1954,
when it was incorporated as a separate, unaffiliated organization. Al-
Anon is a self-help fellowship of men, women, and children whose
lives have been affected by the compulsive drinking of a family
member or friend. Alateen, a part of Al-Anon Family Groups, helps
teenage sons and daughters of alcoholics to cope with problems in
their homes. These groups provide direct services to individuals by
giving comfort, hope, and friendship to the family and friends of
alcoholics, by providing information on alcoholism and sharing
experience in coping with the disease, and by providing the opportunity to learn to grow spiritually."

Co-Dependents Anonymous (CoDA)
P.O. Box 33577, Phoenix, AZ 85067-3577
Phone: (602) 277-7991

"...established in 1986 as a self-help recovery program for individuals coping with codependency. Codependency is a compulsive,
self-destructive behavior, usually caused by dysfunctional family systems. The disorder is characterized by an inability to maintain func-
tional relationships, and may include a history of addiction. CoDA is
a nonprofessional organization, and is not allied with any sect,
denomination, politics, organization, or institution. Its group activities are patterned after twelve-step recovery programs. Group meetings have been established in forty-nine states and ten countries, and
an International Service Conference is held annually in Phoenix."

Families Anonymous (FA)
P.O. Box 3475, Culver City, CA 90231-3475
Phone: (800) 736-9805 or (310) 313-5800; Fax: (310) 313-6841

"...founded in 1971 as a mutual support group for families of people involved in drug abuse and related behavioral problems. Group meetings and discussions are modeled on the twelve steps of Alcoholics Anonymous and focus on providing emotional support for the member rather than changing the behavior of the substance abuser. There are no fees or dues for group membership. Assistance is offered to people forming new FA groups."

Gamblers Anonymous
Information Services Offices
P.O. Box 17173, Los Angeles, CA 90010
Phone: (213) 386-8789

"Gamblers Anonymous, formed in 1957, is a fellowship of men and women who share their experiences, strengths, and hopes with each other in order to solve their common problem and to help others recover from a compulsive gambling problem. The twelve steps used in Alcoholics Anonymous are modified for use in this self-help fellowship. A booklet presenting the basic program is available, and requesters will be referred to the local group nearest them."

Narcotics Anonymous (NA)
Public Information Coordinator, World Services Office, Inc.
P.O. Box 9999, Van Nuys, CA 91409
Phone: (818) 780-3951; Fax: (818) 785-0923

"...a nonprofit, international organization founded in 1953; it was created to help people of all ages, races, religious perspectives, occupations, and lifestyles stop using drugs. There are twenty-two thousand NA groups in over fifty countries...and more than two thousand meetings are held in correctional and treatment facilities...provides and distributes complimentary group starter kits and NA literature upon request.... NA approaches the twelve-step recovery program by focusing on the disease of addiction itself, and not a particular drug. There are no dues or fees for NA services."

Overeaters Anonymous (OA)
World Service Office
P.O. Box 44020, Rio Rancho, NM 87174-4020

"...founded in 1960, is a self-help group of compulsive overeaters, which promotes a lifetime program of action to relieve the obsession of eating compulsively. Compulsive overeating is viewed as a progressive disease, which can be controlled by a twelve-step recovery program adapted from Alcoholics Anonymous. OA provides pamphlets on its program and holds regular local group meetings worldwide, which are open to all compulsive overeaters."

Secular Organizations for Sobriety (SOS)
SOS National Clearinghouse, The Center for Inquiry, West, 5521 Grosvenor Boulevard, Los Angeles, CA 90066
Phone: (310) 821-8430; Fax: (310) 821-2610
E-mail: sosla@loop.com

"...an alternative recovery method for those alcoholics or drug addicts who are uncomfortable with the spiritual content of widely available twelve-step programs. SOS takes a reasonable, secular approach to recovery and maintains that sobriety is a separate issue from religion or spirituality. SOS credits the individual for achieving and maintaining his or her own sobriety, without reliance on any 'Higher Power.' SOS respects recovery in any form regardless of the path by which it is achieved. It is not opposed to or in competition with any other recovery programs. SOS supports healthy skepticism and encourages the use of the scientific method to understand alcoholism."

Sexual Abuse Anonymous (SAA)
P.O. Box 9665, Berkeley, CA 94709

Sexual Abuse Survivors Anonymous (SASA)
P.O. Box 241046, Detroit, MI 48224
Phone: (313) 882-6446

UPDATE:
Since the publication of *Victims No Longer*, I have been told that several of the organizations that I listed there have ceased to exist. They include Looking Up (Maine), P.L.E.A. (New Mexico), and S.A.S.A.M. (Texas).

WALES: (See also listings for England.)

Swansea Incest and Sexual Abuse Helpline
Phone: (01792) 648-805

Provides: Information, counselling, listening and support for adult survivors of sexual child abuse. Serves South Wales. Hours: Thursday 7:30pm–10pm.

ABOUT THE AUTHOR

Mike Lew, M.Ed., a psychotherapist and group therapy leader in the Boston, Mass., area, is codirector of The Next Step Counseling and Training Center. As a cultural anthropologist specializing in the field of culture and personality (psychological anthropology), he worked with Margaret Mead and Colin Turnbull. After further training in counseling psychology, he became a leading expert on recovery from sexual child abuse, particularly issues of male survivors. He has provided workshops for survivors, professional trainings, consultation, and public lectures throughout the United States and Canada and in Europe and Australia. Mike Lew has taught at The City College of New York, Quinnipiac College, The College of New Rochelle, and University of California at Santa Cruz.

His publications include *Victims No Longer: Men Recovering from Incest and Other Sexual Child Abuse* (HarperCollins, 1990). The first book written specifically for men recovering from sexual child abuse, *Victims No Longer* continues to earn praise for both its clinical expertise and compassionate tone, educating survivors and professionals about the recovery process, speaking to the pain, needs, fears and hopes of the adult male survivor. Mike Lew has consulted to the National Institute of Mental Health, National Resource Center on Child Sexual Abuse, Childhelp USA/National Child Abuse Hotline, People Against Sexual Abuse, and many other organizations in the United States and abroad. He has been on the editorial board of the *Journal of Child Sexual Abuse* and the review board of the *Journal of Interpersonal Violence*.

He has appeared on *The Oprah Winfrey Show, Sally Jessy Raphael, People Are Talking*, and many other television and radio programs.

For further information about workshops and professional trainings, or to be added to Mike Lew's mailing list, see the entry for The Next Step Counseling and Training in the Resources section.

Obtain additional copies of
LEAPING UPON THE MOUNTAINS from your local bookseller.

For bulk discount and trade purchases, call North Atlantic Books
at (800) 337-2665 or visit the North Atlantic Web site:
www.northatlanticbooks.com

Individual signed copies can be ordered directly from
Small Wonder Books

ORDER FORM

Price: U.S.$19.95 for each book. All orders must be accompanied by a check or money order in U.S.$ payable to <u>Small Wonder Books</u>.

Shipping:
Within U.S.: Please add U.S. $4 for the first book and U.S. $2
 for each additional book.
International: U.S.$9 for the first book and U.S.$5 for each
 additional book.
Sales Tax: Please add 5% for books shipped to Massachusetts
 addresses.
Send mail orders to: Small Wonder Books
                       P.O. Box 1146
                       Jamaica Plain, MA 02130

Name: _____

Address: _____

City: _____ State: _____

Zip/Postal Code: _____ Country: _____

☐ Please add my name to your mailing list for notificiation of workshops or trainings in my area

☐ Please send copies signed by the author

For further information about Small Wonder Books and the Next Step
Counseling, visit our Web site at:

http://www.abbington.com/smallwonder/index.html

DATE DUE

GAYLORD   PRINTED IN U.S.A.